Praise for
The ULTIMATE Career Guide for Nurses

Cardillo moves the reader along a buffet table of delectable options for building a life-long, satisfying, and dynamic career in nursing. A feast for all nurses, a banquet for nurses with disabilities. I savored every page!

— Donna Carol Maheady, ARNP, EdD
Adjunct Assistant Professor
Christine E. Lynn College of Nursing at Florida Atlantic University
Founder and President of www.ExceptionalNurse.com

Donna's book is filled with easy-to-read, practical tips about how to manage your career. In addition to identifying specific strategies in each chapter, she addresses common challenges with strategies for everyday career management and skills needed to make a career move. This book is a vital resource for all nurses.

— Barbara A. Brunt, RN-BC, MA, MN
Director of Nursing Education and Staff Development
Summa Health System, Akron, OH
President, National Nursing Staff Development Association

Nursing is a wonderful profession with abundant opportunities for varied roles, specialties, areas of focus, and learning throughout a nurse's career. In her new book, Donna Cardillo offers an excellent resource for any nurse, with practical advice and strategies on how to grow and develop as a nurse as well as ideas on how to move into new and different positions. Her easy writing style, supported with real life examples, provides thought-provoking reading and identifies ways for nurses to enhance their satisfaction, influence, and opportunities. This book also includes important information to assist nurses who are contemplating changes at various stages of their careers.

— Judy Shorr, RN, MS, CHCR
President, National Association for Health Care Recruitment
Recruiter, Children's Hospital & Regional Medical Center, Seattle, WA

D1318470

From everyday professional life to major career challenges, Donna Cardillo's definitive book, *The ULTIMATE Career Guide for Nurses,* provides nurses with the tools to examine their own talents, skills, and interests; explore the career landscape; and become empowered to create their own future. Cardillo, a nationally recognized expert on career development for nurses, has specific advice for nurses at any stage in their careers from the novice graduate to the most experienced clinician. This book will become a valued resource, used repeatedly throughout nurses' careers.

— Eleanor J. Sullivan, RN, PhD, FAAN
Author of *Becoming Influential: A Guide for Nurses*
and the Monika Everhardt mysteries
former President, Sigma Theta Tau International

Donna knows nurses and knows what nurses need. She has created a comprehensive guide for staying happy and fulfilled in the profession. Nurses at all stages of their careers will enjoy this book!

— Andrea Higham, Director
The Johnson & Johnson Campaign for Nursing's Future

The ULTIMATE
Career Guide for Nurses
Practical Advice for Thriving at
Every Stage of Your Career

Donna Wilk Cardillo, RN, MA

To Trina —
a great nurse —
Keep making a difference!
Best Wishes —
Donna
Cardillo

Cover Design by Jessica Peterson

Gannett Healthcare Group (publisher of Nurse.com, *Nursing Spectrum, NurseWeek* and *Today in PT*) is a nursing and healthcare communications company and the largest print and electronic publisher of news and information for registered nurses. Our mission is to enrich the professional lives of nurses and other healthcare professionals and to celebrate their unique contributions to society. Our core products include Nurse.com plus 13 regional nursing magazines, an array of award-winning continuing education offerings and more than a dozen annual professional development and nursing specialty guides. Additional products and services include career fairs, web sites, consulting services and an annual television program.

Gannett Healthcare Group
Division of Continuing Education
6400 Arlington Blvd., Suite 1000
Falls Church, VA 22042
(800) 866-0919
ce@gannetthg.com
www.nurse.com

Printed and bound in the United States of America.

ISBN: 978-1-930745-04-9

To my parents, Helen and Stanley Wilk, who passed on all their wonderful talents and traits. You gave me a good foundation in life and then gave me wings to fly.

Contents

Foreword

When you stop to think about it, job-hunting or career development is one of the healing arts. For healing is related to the horizons of our mind.

I used to notice these horizons when I was a parish priest and had to visit three hospitals in my community every day. I noticed that when hospital patients were at death's door, the horizons of their mind had shrunk pretty much to just what was happening with their body that day. And so it would continue. But when they started to get well, they started asking questions or talking about other people in the hospital, then about things going on with their family or friends, then things going on in the community, then the nation, then the world. They started asking for newspapers and magazines. Their minds were pushing outward; their horizons were expanding. They were starting to heal and get well. The two things are intimately related.

As nurses, our routine over the years can become so stifling, humdrum, mind-numbing, or boring that the horizons of our mind also start to shrink. I remember a nurse who said to me: "Home. Hospital. Supermarket. Church. Week after week. This is all there is to my life." We too sometimes need healing.

So, what happens to us when we start to think about our future, as Donna Cardillo recommends in her excellent book here? What happens when we start to examine ourselves and our gifts more fully and imagine other places where we might use those gifts? Well, you know what happens. We start to push out of the horizons of our mind. And the more we push them out, the more the extent of the healing.

As you read this book, think about every step that Donna recommends you take: the lists, the notebook, the self-examination, the accumulating of new experiences, the volunteering, the exploring of career options, and so on. You will notice they all add up to one thing — the pushing out the horizons of your mind and spirit.

This is why I think this kind of exploration should be mandatory for nurses, and the longer you have been in nursing, the more important it is. You're not just doing some selfish meditation about your own future. You are practicing one of the healing arts. You will be a better healer with your patients and everyone around you, as a result.

And — lucky you — in Donna you have the country's leading expert on career development for nurses to guide you.

Richard Bolles, Author
What Color Is Your Parachute?
A Practical Manual For Job-Hunters and Career Changers
The most popular career guide in the world
10,000,000 copies in print, in 20 languages, revised annually

Acknowledgements

So many brilliant, talented, and passionate people contributed in some way to this book. To these individuals, you have my respect, gratitude, admiration, and affection. I am in your debt. I would like to acknowledge:

- Everyone at Gannett Healthcare Group — past and present — for making this book a reality and for allowing me to speak in my own voice. Special thanks to Robert Hess, Dody Angelini, Lisa Foulke, Catherine Wiley, Fred DiCoztanzo, Patti Rager, and Cindy Saver.

- Richard Bolles for his generosity and inspiring and insightful foreword. You honor me and the entire nursing profession with your support. You are The Man!

- Expert contributors and peer reviewers Jeanne Beaugard, Rosemary Farrell, Nancy Dreher, Edward Wilk, Joseph Cardillo, Helen Sanchez, Joan Orseck, Catherine Tansey, Barbara Davis, and Barbara Bastian.

- Those who I interviewed or quoted or who shared stories and experiences, including Patti Rager, Rosemary Farrell, Krystyna Lis, Jacqueline W. Riley, Joan Borgatti, Barbara Shea Tracy, Cathy Gallo, Kathleen Pagana, and countless others with whom I have worked or spoken over the years.

- Barbara Acello for all her help, support, and encouragement in my early writing days.

- My wonderful husband Joe, editorial assistant extraordinaire, a great writer and editor in his own right, gourmet cook, artist, and all around brilliant and talented guy. Did I mention handsome?

- My amazing family, including Helen and Stanley; David, Justyna, Joao, and Sebastian; Pia; Barbara, Barry, and Anna; Ed, Nancy, Mimi, Andrew, and Matthew; Pam, Paul, Lily, and Max; Rose, Eugene, and Linda for your unconditional love and support — not to mention good laughs and good times.

- To all my nursing colleagues who make a positive difference in the world everyday. This project was a labor of love, and you are so worth it.

Introduction

After publishing my first book *Your First Year as a Nurse — Making the Transition From Total Novice to Successful Professional,* nurses have been asking me, "When are you going to write a book for the rest of us that are beyond our first year?" *The ULTIMATE Career Guide for Nurses* is my response.

This book is a compilation of wisdom, insights, and resources accumulated over my 30 plus years in nursing. I devoted the last 14 years to the study and promotion of what makes nurses successful. People define success in different ways, but it all comes down to this: Being happy, fulfilled, inspired, enthusiastic, and always growing, while keeping a sense of passion and purpose. That's what *The ULTIMATE Career Guide for Nurses* is about.

We nurses are very focused on the technical side of our profession: Clinical issues, patient care, and nursing science are all vitally important. What we haven't always focused on is our own personal and professional growth and development. Many of us who have been in nursing for some time never mapped out a career plan for ourselves or had a contingency plan within nursing if things didn't work out as we anticipated. A large number of us never learned or realized the benefits of developing professional goals and networks and creating a sense of community in nursing.

We are also notorious for underestimating or failing to recognize our own value and worth, including the vast body of knowledge and experience we possess even right out of nursing school. Most nurses are not aware of the multitude of opportunities available to them — even in their current place of employment. Nor have we always been effective in leveraging our education and skill set to our best advantage. In other words, we never learned how to, or saw the value of self-promotion, self-marketing, and self-preservation.

Are the altruistic motives of nursing in opposition to career building and self-promotion? On the contrary, they are essential to recruit good candidates into the profession, to keep nurses in the nursing profession, and to support professional development and growth. If nursing is to be defined as a professional career rather than simply a skilled job, we must develop a career path for ourselves as individuals and career standards that support the entire profession.

When I started nursing school more than 30 years ago, I never dreamed that I'd be where I am today: owning my own business, authoring books, speaking all around the world, writing an advice column for nurses, and contributing to the greater good in my own unique way. Nor did I imagine that I would have a series of nursing jobs over the decades that allowed me to contribute to healthcare in a wide variety of ways and places and discovering more about myself and the world around me in the process. What I know now is that nursing is the most diverse profession on the planet. Nursing will take you anywhere you want to go. Getting into nursing was one of the best decisions I ever made and that is why I wrote this book.

Here's to your success, longevity, and sheer joy in nursing. My cap is off to all of you!

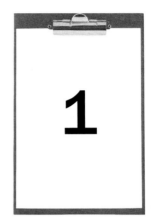

This Profession We Call Nursing

In spite of all the changes in healthcare today, nursing still offers rich and diverse opportunities. For those willing to leave old stereotypes behind, to step outside of their comfort zone, and to avail themselves of all that this glorious profession has to offer, the challenges, rewards, and means for self-actualization and fulfillment are great.

Many nurses believe that nursing is not a job, but a career. What's the difference? A job is simply something you show up for everyday. You put in your hours, go home, and then repeat the cycle the next day. Very little ever changes and your work is routine and mundane. You operate on automatic pilot, resist change, and work to collect a paycheck. You stay in one place until you get bored, fired, or retire. Some people stay with a job even though they're bored or burnt out because of their fear of making changes or their belief that they have no options. They get into a rut and can't seem to get themselves out.

On the other hand, a career is something you plan for and work at. It constantly evolves and expands whether you work in one place or move around during your professional life. A career is like a living, breathing organism that changes and grows over time. It needs continuous nourishment through new experiences, education, risk-taking, and challenges. And while a career requires a solid base, it is pliable enough to adapt to an ever-changing environment.

Career management involves feeding and weeding and constantly reshaping your career landscape. It is a perpetual cycle of renewal and growth, a process of stretching yourself and always moving in a positive forward direction. Managing your career keeps your professional life fresh and active, alive and well. Learning to effectively manage your career will lead to a happier, more fulfilling, and rewarding career. It's the antidote to stagnation that will increase your longevity in this profession. Managing your career puts you in the driver's seat. Nurses have more control over their workplace and professional lives than they realize. They also have more opportunities than they are aware of and possess more skills and abilities, even right out of nursing school, than most give themselves credit for. And while nursing skills are acquired in school, how to manage and nurture a career is often something we must learn on our own.

The components of an effective career management plan include —

- Knowing your industry and keeping abreast of changes
- Knowing yourself through self-assessment and self-awareness
- Developing goals and creating a plan of action
- Taking calculated risks in your career for advancement and growth
- Trying new things and stretching yourself
- Being proactive rather than passive
- Getting into a cycle of continuous formal and informal learning
- Becoming proficient at self-marketing
- Developing professional networks
- Maintaining career mobility
- Achieving a healthy balance between professional and personal lives

Unfortunately, many nurses don't understand the concept of career management. It is not something you do only when looking for a job. Rather, career management is an ongoing activity designed to get the most out of your current job and your career in the long run.

I recently attended a convention where I was representing Nursing Spectrum at its exhibit booth. I was giving out copies of the *Pathways to Professional Development* magazine, an annual career management tool. When offered a complimentary copy, many nurses declined, saying, "No thanks, I'm not looking to change jobs," or "I don't need that; I'm happy where I am." Another began to shake her head back and forth and said, "Oh, no. I've got my heels dug in where I am and will be there until I retire." I found these reactions interesting and amusing as clearly these nurses equated anything to do with career management with changing jobs. The guide contained much more than how to find a job. For example, it had articles about public speaking, self-care for nurses, e-mail etiquette, time management, and how to make the most of meetings. It also addressed usual clinical and nontraditional specialties and even issues such as how to get out of debt and investing. All of these things are elements of an effective career management plan.

The reaction I received at the convention is not uncommon. Many nurses believe that as long as they are employed, all is well. Employment becomes their security blanket, conveying a false sense of stability. They become comfortable and insulated and don't feel the need to stay fully connected to the world around them. It's amazing how many nurses are certain they will never need to look for another job. However, jobs don't last forever, and nurses may not want to or be able to stay in their present jobs in the future. Let's face it, job security is an illusion. Nursing shortage or not, no one is immune to lay-offs, reengineering, mergers, and buy-outs. Here are a few other situations to consider: What if you became disabled or developed a back or shoulder injury? What if you decided to go back to school and needed a flexible schedule, or simply wanted a different lifestyle at some point? These are realities of life and work to think about.

I recently spoke with a long-time OR nurse. In the course of conversation, I asked her if she had ever thought of what she would do if she ever decided to leave the OR. She quickly responded, "Oh that will never happen. I love what I do, and people will always need surgery." I reminded her that while people will always need some type of surgery in our lifetime, more and more surgery is being done on an outpatient basis. New technology is fueling less invasive procedures. And fewer people need certain types of surgery because of more sophisticated diagnostics. One nurse told me that a multihospital system recently purchased her hospital and all of the employees had to reapply for their own jobs. Here's another scenario: Things may be just fine where you are now until a new manager or administrator is hired and everything changes. One thing is guaranteed — your job is going to change, whether you stay where you are or not.

If you're happy in your current position, looking to make a change, exploring your options for the future, or just wanting to take your career to the next level, career management should be a part of everything you do. If you are not actively managing your career, then you can't very well complain about your circumstances.

What Is a Nurse?

When asked what we do, many nurses lapse into industry jargon about performing assessments, administering medications, monitoring health status, and other similar things. But nursing is less about the tasks we perform and more about a knowledge-based practice that plays a key role in every aspect of healthcare.

What is a nurse? A nurse is a combination of education, experiences, skills, abilities, and the capacity to care and to give. We as nurses are not defined by where we work or whether or not we wear a uniform or scrubs to work. It is about who we are. Nurses are vital at the bedside, but we are just as vital in every other aspect of the healthcare arena. We have been making a difference in many ways and places since the beginning of our profession.

What do nurses do? We promote health and wellness. We facilitate entry into this life and departure from it. We touch lives and we save lives. We bring light into dark places. Nurses are teachers, nurturers, and healers. The world has always needed a lot of healing — of the mind, body, spirit, and self-esteem. We are caregivers, patient advocates, researchers, educators, lobbyists, change agents, managers, administrators, and counselors. And sometimes we are simply another human being sharing in the experience of life and death.

Being a nurse is not something you turn on and off. Nurses are never off duty. If someone in our family or in our circle of friends gets sick or needs healthcare advice, we are on. We are vigilant to the health needs of the world. Even today as a nurse entrepreneur traveling the world, speaking, writing, and coaching, I am a health advisor and educator, telephone triage nurse, bereavement counselor, first-aid provider, home care nurse, and care planner and coordinator for my extended family and friends. Once a nurse, always a nurse.

Nurses do many different things in many different places. One of the great things about this profession is an endless opportunity to meet each nurse's interests, special skills, scheduling needs, physical ability, and location. There is never a reason to be bored. However, the general public, and even some nurses, have a deeply entrenched view that nurses work almost exclusively at the bedside in a traditional role. When you tell people you're a nurse, often the first thing they ask is, "What hospital do you work in?" The moment I stepped out of the hospital years ago into a nontraditional nursing role, people would ask me why I left nursing. Some nurses even still think that those who work in nontraditional roles are not real nurses, a view that frames us in a limited capacity. It serves to box us in and confines us to one specific role and work setting. This perception views nurses as one-dimensional. Then when we try to get out into the world to be visible, vocal, and taken seriously, people want to know what we're doing outside of the hospital. That mentality makes people wonder what a woman is doing outside of the kitchen.

Some people fear that nurses would be lured away from bedside nursing if they knew about nontraditional options, as if keeping nurses in the dark is the way to keep them at the bedside. On the contrary, many nurses truly love bedside nursing and wouldn't do anything else. In fact, some nurses who had left the workforce or had taken on administrative or nontraditional roles are now looking to return to bedside nursing. For them, bedside care is nursing at its best because that's where the action is and their hearts are.

Some nurses do need or want a less physically demanding environment, have specific scheduling needs, or simply wish to put their knowledge and skills to work in a different way than the bedside. While I do not encourage anyone to leave the hospital setting, I suggest that we need to embrace an expanded view of who we are and what we do as a profession. It's time to celebrate the variety within nursing. It's time to revel in our accomplishments and contributions, whether at the bedside or in the boardroom, whether doing research or calibrating IV pumps, whether dressed in pumps and pearls, or scrubs and clogs. We are all in the same profession trying to make an impact, trying to make positive changes, and doing our part. And although we are all different people, we share one heart, one soul, and one voice as nurses.

Am I still a nurse today, as a writer, speaker, and career coach? You'd better believe it. I am just as much a nurse standing in front of an audience in a business suit, or sitting at my computer in jeans as I was when I wore a white uniform and cap and worked in the ED. I am still a teacher, nurturer, and healer in everything I do. I just do it in a different way. My philosophy, values, and mission haven't changed. I have no doubt that I am still contributing to the greater good of healthcare. I am a nurse first and a business owner second. Once a nurse, always a nurse.

Changing Times

As the world around us is changing, healthcare and nursing is changing, too. While many nurses groan about managed care being responsible for all that ails us in healthcare today, managed care did not create many of the changes we see. Rather, the concept of managed care surfaced in an effort to address rapidly rising costs and a sudden drain on finances and other resources in healthcare.

For starters, the population is rapidly aging. We're all living longer and even though as we age, we're healthier and more active than previous generations, the older we get, the more healthcare services we need. According to the Administration on Aging, a division of the U.S. Department of Health and Human Services, people older than 65 had about four times the number of days of hospitalization as did those younger than 65 in 2000. Older persons averaged almost twice as many contacts with physicians in 2000 than persons of all ages.

Because of continuously escalating costs in healthcare, we are constantly looking for innovative ways to deliver good quality, cost-effective healthcare. This search has shifted care from traditional hospitals to the home, community, and other alternate care settings, including subacute care, rehabilitation, and long-term care. Hospital care is expensive and is an often less than ideal setting for meeting the healthcare needs of many populations. Patients who do come into the hospital may be sicker, but stay for a shorter period of time.

A boom in technology has facilitated the development of computers in healthcare to test, diagnose, and in some cases, even treat and monitor patients from remote locations. Computers also allow us to keep better records and manage the flow of information. They are great tools for education and research. We continue to see advances in medical and nursing practice and research. Significant progress has been made in the areas of transplantation, genetic engineering, and the manufacture of artificial body parts and human organs, such as skin and corneas, which are now being grown in the lab. We have better diagnostics and treatment modalities, less invasive procedures, and more effective drugs.

The traditional healthcare community, including managed care companies, has shifted the past focus on acute illness to staying well and managing chronic illness. Western medicine is beginning to embrace holistic practices and philosophies that focus on the whole person rather than a specific disease process. Our society is looking for more natural solutions for staying well and healing. Perhaps we're getting tired of being poked, prodded, and medicated.

We've also seen a resurgence of spirituality and a reemerging sense of community. On the downside, we're living in an increasingly violent society plagued not only by global terrorism, but by local issues of domestic violence, child and elder abuse, and sexual abuse and assault. More of these events are reported these days, and more victims are coming forward for treatment and justice.

These industrial and societal changes have made way for new, exciting specialties in nursing. For example, forensic nursing is now a bona fide nursing specialty, combining nursing science with law enforcement. In this specialty, nurses might work with victims of sexual assault or on cases of suspected elder or child abuse. Some forensic nurses investigate deaths for medical examiners, while others even serve as coroners.

Faith community nursing is a new specialty born of the trend to bring healthcare back into the community and to reconnect with spirituality in our lives. Faith community nurses work in conjunction with religious congregations to provide healthcare services similar to those delivered by public health nurses, while offering spiritual support as well. Likewise, more and more nurses are getting involved in chaplaincy programs in healthcare facilities.

Nursing informatics has emerged to combine nursing science with computer science. Informatics nurses work for healthcare facilities and information technology companies managing and interpreting patient care data, coordinating computerized patient charting systems, consulting on the development of software to be used by nurses, and acting as educators, trouble shooters, and facilitators in the process.

Holistic nursing is experiencing a boon. And while some would say that nurses have always practiced holistically, nurses have taken holistic health and wellness to a new level. Many nurses are certified in modalities such as massage therapy, Reiki, therapeutic touch, and aromatherapy. Some nurses incorporate holistic nursing principles and practice into their bedside practice or become independent practitioners in this field.

These are just a few examples of new and emerging specialties in nursing in response to changing times. The nursing profession is constantly changing, evolving, and adapting as things around us change and as we continue to expand our own vision of who we are, what we are capable of doing, and how we fit into the system.

What Else Has Changed?

Not so long ago, the profile of the typical nursing student was a young woman right out of high school. Most attended hospital-based training programs, and few went on to higher education. All that has changed. Findings of the National Sample Survey of Registered Nurses conducted by the Health Resources and Service Administration indicate that between 1980 and 2004 the percentage of nurses who received their basic education in diploma programs decreased from 63% to 25% of the RN population. During that same timeframe, those who received their basic education in associate's degree programs increased from 19% to 42%. The percentage receiving that education from baccalaureate programs increased from 17% to 30%. In addition, an estimated 0.5% of RNs in 2004 had received their initial nursing education through a master's or doctoral degree program.

Likewise, more licensed nurses now go on to further their education. For example, according to the same study, the majority of all licensed nurses in 1980 listed a high school diploma as their highest level of education. In 2004, that had changed with highest education being an associate degree for 33%, a baccalaureate degree for 34%, and a master's degree for 13%. Although the presence of men (5%) and minorities (11%) still represents a small percentage of overall RNs, the data shows that those numbers are also increasing.

More and more people are coming into nursing as a second, third, or fourth career. Therefore, many students are older and bring diverse work experience with them into nursing. These "multi-careerists" come to the profession with degrees in other disciplines. All of these elements will only serve to strengthen nursing in the future.

Some new graduates are going directly into advanced practice. They either come out of school as nurse practitioners (NP) or enter the nursing profession with the intent of becoming a certified registered nurse anesthetist (CRNA) or certified nurse midwife (CNM) after obtaining prerequisite experience. Some nurses say, "That's not good. You have to practice at a basic level first before going into advanced practice." But who says you can't start out at a basic level as an advanced practice nurse? We have to be open to new ways of thinking and of doing things. There would be no progress without that. Nothing stays the same. We have to move forward.

Why are people coming into nursing today? Most men and women come to nursing for the same altruistic reasons that nurses of past generations did. A lot of people came into nursing during the last shortage looking for a job and good pay. But some of them who may not have previously considered nursing are taking a second look at it. Some multi-careerists have become disillusioned with the corporate world, especially in light of the recent rash of corporate corruption and greed that have dominated the headlines, and want to do something more meaningful with their lives and careers. Also, the spotlight on the helping professions as a result of terrorism and other tragic events in our lives has brought to light the important role that nurses play in healthcare. And, of course, a booming job market with ever-expanding opportunities, including advanced practice roles, doesn't hurt either.

One Nurse's Journey

I can't recall the exact moment I decided to become a nurse, but I remember developing a love affair with the profession early on. I always loved science, and I couldn't think of any area more interesting than human science. While in high school, I worked as a candy striper in a hospital and felt energized by the fast-paced human drama that surrounded me. I remember the sense of awe I experienced while entering the inner sanctum of the intensive care unit (ICU) with dinner trays. I remember the excitement and joy of walking past the nursery window and seeing all that new life squirming and fussing. I remember the emotion in the voices of family members and friends who would call for information about the status of their loved ones. I recall how my heart would beat faster when an ambulance sped down the street and into the ED driveway. I can still see all the important looking people walking around with a sense of purposefulness on their faces. And most of all, I remember the patients.

I used to love to watch old hospital movies and fell in love with the image of the nurse — the starched white uniform, the cap, the sensible lace-up oxford shoes. In fact, once I was accepted into nursing school, I was so eager to own a pair of nursing shoes that a good friend gave me my first pair of Clinic© shoes as a high school graduation gift. She couldn't have given me anything better. I should have had those shoes bronzed. They were so symbolic to me. Little did I know at the time all the miles and all the places those shoes, and subsequent pairs, would take me in this glorious profession.

On the journey, I began to learn that people who are not nurses often do not understand what the profession is all about and what we get out of it. They often say, "I could never do what you do," or "I don't know how you do it." Outsiders see only the challenges and hardships, such as dealing with human pain and suffering, working long hours, and dealing with difficult people. What nonnurses could not possibly see or know is the overwhelming sense of contributing to the greater good, of making a difference in the lives of others, of being there for people during their darkest and most vulnerable hours, of impacting the health and wellness of the population. It's difficult to explain the feeling we get when someone looks into our eyes and even without words says, "Thank you." Or when someone who wasn't expected to live or walk again somehow recovers and goes home largely as a result of good nursing care and support. It is the reward of care giving.

I also found that a common misunderstanding people who aren't nurses have is that nurses are somehow a rung or two below physicians in the healthcare chain. Every nurse has been asked at one time or another in his or her career, "Gee, you're so intelligent. Why didn't you become a doctor?" implying that intelligent people become doctors and not-so-intelligent people become nurses. Because the profession has always been predominantly female, I sometimes hear people say that women did not have many career

"Why Didn't You Become a Doctor?"

Jackie says, *"The best response I ever heard was, 'Why on earth would I want to be an MD? I have the best possible position [as a nurse] for getting to know and helping people over the long term.'"*

choices in the past and that's why many chose nursing when they were younger. What they fail to realize is that many of us knew we had options and believed we could be whatever we wanted to be. And still we made a deliberate, conscious, and enlightened choice to go into nursing. I was born to be a nurse. There is nothing else that I would do, even today. Nursing has been the ride of my life.

When I started out almost 30 years ago, like many nurses, I had only images of nurses at the bedside. I presumed that was what I would always do. A modern-day Florence Nightingale, that was me. During nursing school, I had an opportunity to work part-time as an electrocardiograph (ECG) technician. That experience introduced me to the ED. I spent a great deal of time there and was intrigued by the fast pace, the diversity of cases, and the precision with which everyone seemed to work. It was almost like watching a ballet with beautifully choreographed movements, crescendos, and diminuendos. I later worked in the ED as a nurse's aide while a student nurse and grew to love it.

I had some great psychiatric nursing instructors in school who were so enthusiastic about the specialty that I developed a keen interest in it. So, while a student, I also worked in a county psychiatric hospital, which was home to many chronically mentally ill men and women. Many of the patients I encountered there had been abandoned long ago by family members or had simply outlived their relatives and had nowhere else to go. This environment was so different from the ED of a community hospital in an affluent neighborhood and offered very unique challenges. In the ED, patients came and went quickly. We treated and released people or stabilized them before moving them out to another department. In the county psychiatric facility, I had the opportunity to develop long-standing relationships with patients and learn about their families, histories, and backgrounds. I was already discovering the diversity that the profession had to offer me. Needless to say, both environments were eye opening for me.

Upon graduation, there were no openings in the ED where I worked as a student, so I initially worked in another facility that offered extensive psychiatric services. I chose to work on a locked ward for male patients. As a new nurse, I was ready to take on some challenges. This unit served as an admission ward for those with addictive disorders, those with court-ordered 72-hour admissions, county prisoners who required psychiatric evaluation, and any other acute psychiatric admissions. Here I began to better understand the complexities of the human mind. I encountered patients with significant substance abuse problems, people accused of violent crimes, those from abusive and dysfunctional homes, individuals who were severely depressed, homeless people, and various others with acute and chronic mental illness. Some nurses have an aversion to psychiatric nursing, and yet I found it to be one of the most fascinating and challenging specialties.

Although I loved psychiatric nursing, my heart was in the ED. So when I heard about an opening in my old department, I grabbed the opportunity. The ED exposed me to the full spectrum of the human experience on a moment-to-moment basis. Even though I was working in a small community hospital, I saw my share of trauma and other medical and surgical emergencies. I also saw many patients with run-of-the-mill minor medical complaints and chronic illness, those who didn't have a family physician, or thought it was easier to come to the ED. This was, of course, in the days before managed care. I even assisted with the occasional birth of an overly eager baby in a car in the ED driveway.

Why Choose Nursing?

One nurse's recollection about choosing nursing as a profession many years ago:

"I remember my aunt, who was an author, telling me I could 'do better than that' and be a doctor or a writer, as I so love to write. She would often say, 'Why be just a nurse? You're wasting yourself in such a lowly profession.'

"But you know, when she was dying of breast cancer almost three years ago, I stayed at her house with her (she lived alone) for her last two weeks. I felt honored to be able to be there as her favorite niece...and, as her nurse. The night before she died, she said: 'What would I do without you? Thank God you're a nurse.' This was the last thing she said to me. I still get a heart tug every time I remember this."

— Barb

In the ED, I developed a true appreciation for the sacredness and fragility of human life. I loved the ED because I was exposed to many specialties: cardiac, obstetrics (OB), pediatrics, orthopedics, neurology, and psychiatry. Of course, because of my mental-health background and their psychiatric nursing phobia, my coworkers assigned the psychiatric patients to me.

My ED doubled as the outpatient department for the hospital. That meant we ran outpatient clinics for all specialties and performed procedures like colonoscopies, blood transfusions, and minor surgery. We were also a poison-control center, and ran public-screening programs for diabetes, mouth cancer, eye health, and other services. There was very little I wasn't exposed to in that ED, one way or another.

At the time, I presumed I would always work as an ED nurse because that's who I was, that's what I did. But then I got married and bought a house far from where I was working. I had to leave my beloved ED to look for employment in a new location. Of course, I thought I would just find another job in an ED in my new neck of the woods because that's who I was, and that's what I did. I began to scan the classified ads, since that was the only way I knew to look for a job at the time. Although I saw some ED positions advertised, they were almost all for the evening or night shift. That was not conducive to my lifestyle as a newlywed.

Expanding My Horizons

When I couldn't find a day job in an ED, I began to explore other options. I noticed an ad for a part-time job in a medical weight-control center. I needed a full-time job, but I was intrigued by the position and wanted to learn more. Besides, I figured maybe I'd have access to some of their secrets and actually lose a few pounds if I worked there! I picked up the phone and made an appointment for an interview. After the usual questions and answers about the job, the nurse conducting the interview said, "Would you by any chance be interested in a full-time position?" I agreed enthusiastically. She continued, "It just so happens we have a head nurse position open in a center in your area. Would you consider that?" "Yes," I replied having no idea what I was in for next. With that, she escorted me down the hall to meet with the president of the company. I was totally unprepared for this. I thought I would breeze in, get a little information, and go on my merry way. I hadn't even dressed that well because I had interviewed more out of curiosity than a belief that I would receive a job offer of any kind.

I was now in the inner sanctum of the executive offices of this company, dressed way too casually, and feeling scared and overwhelmed. I was introduced to the company president, and he began asking me real interview questions, such as, "What are your goals?" I don't believe I had any goals back then. I was in a state of panic because as a nurse, I never had an actual interview in my life. Years ago, interviews for nurses consisted of one question, "When can you start?" All of this aside, as a nurse, I was accustomed to thinking on my feet. And like many nurses, I was more intelligent than I gave myself credit for at the time. I answered his questions as best I could and apparently did OK because at the end of the interview he said, "Well, congratulations. You have the job!" Bewildered, I asked, "Well, excuse me, but which job do I have?" I was so confused at that point. The company president responded, "The head nurse position!" I thought it was pretty good that I applied for a part-time staff position and left with a full-time management position.

Was this a fluke? Not at all. It has happened to many nurses before and after me. In fact, this sort of thing happens all the time when you get out there and interview. I had applied to what is known as an open job, one that is publicly advertised and usually has many competing applicants. I left with what is known as a hidden job, an opening that exists in a company that is not publicly advertised. Hidden jobs account for the majority of available jobs out there. I learned a valuable lesson: An interview is always an opportunity.

Looking back, this was a perfect transitional position for me. I was expected to work in my white uniform and cap (this was in the 1970s) and would be drawing blood and taking ECGs, so I still felt like a "real nurse." I learned a lot about nutrition and the mechanics of weight loss and gain, including physiological and psychological factors. I counseled and taught patients and offered lots of support. I was also learning a little about the business side of healthcare. And for those of you who are wondering, I did lose some weight while I worked there, but I gained it all back after I changed jobs!

Just a Nurse?

About 10 months into my new job, the company president asked to have lunch with me. I was a little nervous, but knew that I was thought well of in the company and felt confident that I was doing a good job. Shortly into lunch he blurted out, "The manager in your center is being transferred to another location, and I'd like you to take over managing that center." I was dumbstruck. If I had been swallowing food at that moment, I would have needed the Heimlich maneuver. I broke out into a cold sweat and began to stutter and sputter and flail my arms as I proclaimed in a high-pitched voice, "I can't do that. I'm just a nurse!" To further my point I added, "I don't know anything about personnel issues, advertising, selling, or management. Thanks, but no thanks." I presumed I had effectively put an end to his absurd notion.

With a slight smile on his face, the businessman sat there considering my reaction, and what I had just said. I couldn't imagine what he found amusing. Finally, he said very emphatically, "I understand your reluctance, but I think you can do the job. I want you to take it." In essence, he wasn't giving me a choice. I had once heard that if you are offered a promotion on the job and you don't accept it, you might not have much of a future with that company. For that reason alone, I reluctantly accepted the position of center manager.

· ·

Being a nurse is not something you turn on and off.

· ·

Once the decision was made, I experienced panic I had never felt before. Maybe it wasn't as bad as when I had to give my first injection to a person rather than a navel orange, or the time I found myself alone in a psychiatric ward with a 6'5" 350-pound psychotic man who had just thrown a chair through a window, or the time... OK, OK, I think I made my point. Let's just say that I spent a miserable, sleepless weekend wondering what I had gotten myself into. I lost respect for this man. How could he put someone like me in charge of one of his business ventures? What was he thinking? I figured it would probably take me three to six months to completely run the business into the ground. It would just be a matter of time before I was pounding the pavement again, looking for work. No one was more convinced than I that I would fail miserably in this new position.

As if that wasn't enough, I now had to wear street clothes to work, and I didn't have any. I had a typical nurse's wardrobe — white uniforms and casual clothes. I did have a fancy dress in case I had to go to a wedding or other festive event, but that dress usually didn't fit me the second time I needed it anyway. I had no idea what to wear to work unless it was white and sold in a uniform store.

The big day finally arrived. I threw together an outfit, took a few deep breaths, and told myself I'd been in tougher spots than this. For instance, there was that time in the ED when... you get my gist. An amazing thing happened once I started in my new position. Slowly but surely, like everything else in life, I began to learn what I needed to know to manage that center. I learned by asking questions, by doing, by observing experienced people, by trial and error, and sometimes just by figuring things out on my own, which nurses are very good at. In fact, I learned it all so well that eight months later, the owner of the company asked me to open and manage a second center for him. By now, I had the management thing down pat, so I said, "No problem." I had certainly come a long way, and I began to fully appreciate all the skills and attributes I possessed as a nurse.

Let me assure you that in comparison to what we have learned in nursing school and during our practice, acquiring business skills is easy. However, because it is different from what we are accustomed to, we might assume we can't do it. But how often have you encountered a new procedure or piece of equipment or been pulled to work in an unfamiliar unit? You always adapt, learn what you need to, and find a way to get the job done. It's the same thing here. But take a nurse out of the hospital, and that nurse often forgets what he or she is capable of. Nurses are smart. I know this because we need to be to get through nursing school, pass a rigorous state licensing exam, and to do what we do every day. We are also multitalented and versatile, qualities in ourselves that we often miss.

As you can imagine, managing two centers was a 24-hour-a-day, seven-day-a-week responsibility. After working at this company for several years, my personal circumstances changed. I was now looking for something that was strictly 9 AM to 5 PM, Monday through Friday, and low stress. The ideal job, right? I even wanted something close to home so I could walk to work if needed. Again, I began combing the classified ads looking for something different and, hopefully, interesting. I saw an ad for a part-time staff position in an office that did medical exams for insurance companies. They were not even looking for a nurse, but the work sounded intriguing and the office was a few blocks from where I lived. I needed a full-time job, but decided to go on the interview anyway. During the interview, the woman asked, "Would you by any chance be interested in a full-time position?" I gleefully replied, "Yes. Actually, I need a full-time job." She responded, "It just so happens that our office manager is getting married and moving out of state. Would you be interested in that position?" I could hardly believe this was happening for the second time. Now that I had some management experience under my belt, I eagerly told her I was interested.

With that, she brought me in to meet the franchise owner. At least I had dressed better this time. I learned my lesson the first time around. At the end of the interview, I was offered the position of office manager. The salary was much lower than what I had been making in the weight control center, but I was so desperate to make a change I accepted the position and figured I'd find a way to make ends meet. At that point in time, my work situation was more important to me than the money. Don't get me wrong; I needed the money. I just needed my sanity and a regular schedule more.

Once again, I applied to an "open job" and left with a "hidden job." In both positions, I had applied for a part-time staff position and left the interview with a full-time management position. Is this because I was lucky and just in the right place at the right time? I don't believe so. You have to be open to all possibilities as they present themselves. Sometimes you have to take a chance and go on an interview, even if you're not sure what's involved. A one-inch classified ad, or even a large display ad, never tells you everything there is to know about a position, an employer, or the other opportunities that may be waiting in the wings. Once again, this experience illustrates how an interview is always an opportunity.

In this new position, I had to take incoming phone calls from insurance agents about life insurance policies they sold. I determined what the medical requirements of their own company were for issuing the policy and assigned the case to one of our medical field examiners. These examiners were nurses, chiropractors, emergency medical technicians, and other healthcare workers. They went to the person's home or office, completed a medical history, and checked vital signs. I then reviewed these histories for clarity, completeness, and accuracy. Keep in mind that my employer had not used nurses in my position before. He used to train laypeople to do these reviews. However, as a nurse, I picked up inconsistencies or things that needed clarification on these exams that only a person with a healthcare background could detect. He was impressed with my knowledge and was getting compliments from the insurance agents on the accuracy and completeness of the exams. I got my first raise shortly thereafter.

While working for this company, revolutionary changes were taking place in healthcare reimbursement. The Diagnostic Related Groups (DRG) system was introduced in the U.S., which would eventually replace the old itemized billing method. This complex and then controversial system required categorizing inpatients based on their admitting diagnosis along with other medical conditions and treatment factors. Code numbers were assigned to elements in the patient's medical record. This categorization and coding would determine how much reimbursement the hospital would get for that patient's care.

The parent company of the franchise I was working for decided to expand their business and start doing hospital bill auditing and DRG coding verification. Because I was one of the few nurses that were employed by this national company, they asked if they could train me in the DRG system and have me go out on a few calls to hospitals on a trial basis. Of course, always being open to learning something new, I said yes. To be honest, it was also an excuse for me to get away from my usual routine in the office. Little did I know at that time how valuable this experience would be.

All of this ultimately led me to one of the best jobs I had in healthcare — the director of DRG services in a community hospital. This was in the 1980s when hospitals were hiring DRG coordinators to manage the rapidly changing regulatory and reimbursement issues coming down from insurance companies, government, and other agencies. My new employer was looking for a nurse who had familiarity with reimbursement issues. The job was tailor made for me. Additionally, I'd be back working in a hospital, on my home turf so to speak, which made me happy.

What made it even more exciting was that this was a brand new position. I would be responsible for building the department from scratch. I had my own office and was considered part of the management team, reporting directly to hospital, not nursing, administration. That was a big change for me — and an eye-opening one. I had officially become what other nurses have dubbed a member of the "pearls and pumps" group, those of us who wear business suits to work.

Keep in mind that I got the previous job, which led me to this challenging, prestigious position, by applying for a part-time staff position where they weren't even looking for a nurse and were not paying a great starting salary. You never know where the road will take you when you allow yourself to venture out into the world and step outside of your comfort zone.

After that, I worked for a managed care company as the health services manager and later worked for an education company that provided review courses to help nurses pass their state licensing exams. With each new position, I learned something new about myself and about the healthcare industry. I'm still learning as I continue on my journey.

Nursing is a very specific career choice — one filled with challenges, rewards, endless options, and pathways to follow. Nurses are versatile and multitalented. We are vital at the bedside, but we are just as vital in every aspect of the healthcare arena. And just as things around us are constantly changing, so must each of us grow and evolve and keep moving forward to fully take advantage of all that nursing has to offer and to reach our full potential as human beings and as professionals. So let's discuss how you can maximize your opportunities and find happiness and fulfillment in this profession we call nursing.

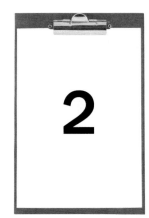

Everyday Career Management

Now that we've established that every nurse should be engaged in career management on an ongoing basis, let's discuss the basics. Obviously, you need to complete specific tasks if you're looking for another job, want to change specialties, or have your sights set on moving up the corporate ladder. But all nurses should maintain basic aspects of their career regardless of their current situation. Let's talk about building a foundation first and move forward from there.

Join a Professional Association

Joining and becoming active in professional associations is a key element of professional success. These organizations hold many opportunities for personal and professional development and growth. They are an essential part of ongoing career management. You cannot develop a career in a vacuum, and that's exactly what you're trying to do if you don't join and get active in your professional associations.

Professional associations provide a forum for disseminating information, providing education, and lending support. They function as a collective voice for people who have common interests and concerns. At the same time, they allow the exchange of ideas among members with diverse opinions. If you think everyone in an association is of one mind, you haven't been out to any meetings lately.

Professional associations are invaluable resources for every nurse from student to retiree. While some well-meaning people encourage nurses to join their professional associations merely out of support for that organization, that is not the best reason to join. You should join because of the personal and professional benefits and opportunities. Here are some examples of what's in it for you.

Membership has its rewards. By joining a professional organization, you become part of a group that forges immediate bonds with other members. If you call or e-mail other members or run into them somewhere, camaraderie arises just from the affiliation, even if you don't otherwise know one another. You have a sense of belonging and being part of a greater whole. And professional associations are some of the best places to find role models, coaches, and mentors.

There are other rewards of membership:

- You start getting related print and electronic publications — local, statewide, and maybe even national. This is one of the best ways to stay on the cutting edge of the most current knowledge and information about your profession and specialty. You'll find out about upcoming educational and networking events, learn about legislative issues that may affect your practice and license, and be in the know on other key industry topics.

- You have a resource whenever you need information, referrals, or answers to questions about your profession. Whether your concerns are clinical, ethical, legal, or simply career-related, you can just pick up the phone or send an e-mail for a timely, expert response or at least a good referral.

- You become entitled to benefits and features reserved for members only. For example, some organizations offer exclusive career services or specialty committees and caucuses for advanced practice, nursing informatics, and other special interests. Many associations offer scholarships, support groups, and in some cases, financial support during illness or hard times. You might get access to special areas of the association's website, such as online advice, continuing education (CE) offerings, chat rooms and bulletin boards, and specialty-specific information, such as salary surveys, demographics, and industry trends.

- You gain a competitive edge that nonmembers may not have. For one thing, the affiliation looks good on your résumé. Memberships in professional associations show that you are an involved and informed professional. This appearance can make a difference when changing jobs, seeking a promotion or transfer, or being considered for other positions and opportunities both inside and outside of your place of employment.

- You have access to powerful and influential people. Because most industry leaders belong to their professional associations, you'll get to rub elbows with the best and the brightest in your profession. That alone can be inspiring. And when people outside the organization are looking for nurses to interview, spotlight, appoint to a government committee or task force, or speak at an event, they often turn to professional associations first.

- You'll receive member discounts to conventions, CE and special programs, and other products and services.

Go to a meeting. By attending the meetings of your professional associations, you'll have an opportunity to meet nurses from other facilities, specialties, and roles. These gatherings are great opportunities to mix and mingle. They provide a forum for sharing information and ideas and finding out what's happening in other places of employment. Not only can you pick up some ideas to bring back to your own department, but you gain perspective on the work world beyond your own job. You can't get a sense of whether things at your workplace are typical or not if you don't know what's happening in other workplaces.

Consider the other benefits of attendance —

- You have an outlet to let off some steam. Many of us don't take time to socialize with our colleagues and have fun. We isolate ourselves and foster a sense of being alone. Even if things are less than ideal where you work, it's comforting to know that others are in the same boat. You can commiserate and even laugh about your common situation, taking comfort in knowing that others share your experience. And attending professional association meetings can be a good excuse to get out of the house for a while.

- You'll always learn something new, either from a CE presenter, an exhibitor, or another meeting participant. And you'll meet some of the most interesting people you'll ever encounter.

Find a committee, be a joiner. By participating in a committee, you'll gain maximum benefit from your membership. You get out of any organization what you put into it. Join a committee that interests you or one where you can develop your special talents. Want to learn more about legislative issues, lobbying, or policy development? Join the political action committee (PAC). Interested in teaching and speaking? Join the education committee. Have an inclination toward writing or marketing? Get on the newsletter or public relations committee. If event planning is something you love to do, volunteer to work on the annual convention or a fundraising project.

There are two other benefits derived from committee work:

- You gain more visibility within the organization when you become active. People get to know you better and vice versa. And for those of you who are shy about meeting new people, this is a great way to overcome your shyness.

- As a committee member, you'll have the opportunity to hone your communication, negotiation, and conflict management skills. You may even learn about finances, marketing, and budgeting. You'll gain experience working with a group and develop your leadership skills.

Don't miss live events. By attending annual conventions and special programs, you become enlightened, energized, and empowered. Conventions, legislative days, and special educational programs are great ways to stay connected to peers and industry leaders on a broader scale. There are always local and statewide events to attend. If you haven't been out to a national convention or meeting in a while, you don't know what you're missing. The experience of meeting colleagues from all over the country is unparalleled. You find out just how similar nurses from different regions are.

Here are just a few added advantages of attending events:

- You'll gain access to industry leaders, such as editors, authors, administrators, educators, researchers, clinicians, and association leaders. I almost always attend my state nurses association convention because anybody who's anybody in the nursing profession in my home state is usually at that convention. There's nothing like meeting notables in person, having an opportunity to shake their hands and having some face time with them.

- You'll have the opportunity to speak with exhibitors from other places of employment, schools of higher education, professional associations, and businesses that offer products and services for nurses and other healthcare professionals. It's a great way to get a lot of information in one place and stay abreast of what's happening in your industry and specialty.

- You'll have an opportunity to attend keynote presentations, educational sessions, and workshops, and pick up some CE credits while doing it. I guarantee you'll come back home with ideas, information, renewed enthusiasm, and new friends.

Buy a ticket to an awards ceremony. By attending awards dinners and galas, you are reminded of all the incredible things nurses do every day to make a difference. It also highlights what is possible to achieve. These events are a celebration of nursing. With all the negative images and messages about nursing today, attending awards ceremonies is one way to reinforce the power and passion of nursing. Regardless of what you do in nursing, seeing your colleagues honored gives you a sense of pride, inspiring and renewing your faith in the profession. Such events remind you what nursing is all about and why you got into the profession in the first place. Listening to the wonderful accomplishments of others can give you something to work toward.

Go the extra mile by seeking an elected position. By running for office, you are forced to step outside of your comfort zone and stretch yourself. The experience builds character, whether you are elected or not. It's also a great opportunity for visibility within the organization.

If you're successful, your position can provide one more reason to interact with other members. One shy colleague of mine once told me that she felt much more comfortable introducing herself to others in the organization because of her elected position. For example, she would introduce herself by saying, "Hi. I'm Janet Rivers, the vice president of programming." She felt that her position gave her the status and confidence to initiate conversations that would have been difficult for her otherwise.

An added benefit of elected office in a professional organization is the impression it can make on current and prospective employers. It demonstrates that you have leadership skills, that you hold the respect of your peers, and that you are a person who can get things done. It looks good on your résumé, too. Holding office in a professional association carries more weight and influence than people realize.

Usual Objections to Not Joining Professional Associations

Some nurses have created an extensive litany of unworthy excuses for nonparticipation in their professional organization. Seasoned by time, but unable to stand up to the scrutiny of a moment, they wonder about the following:

I don't have time to get out to meetings. No one has much free time these days, but we all make time for those things that are important to us. The education, the support, the camaraderie, and the "fun factor" discovered at meetings will be beneficial to you and your career. You'll also develop your social skills. Even if you can't get out to meetings regularly, you'll still have all the other privileges and benefits of membership.

The dues are too expensive. Cost is relative to value. I guarantee you'll get more than your money's worth if you avail yourself of all the association has to offer. Besides, your dues are probably tax-deductible, so talk with your accountant about that. Some associations have special rates or payment plans for students, new graduates, retirees, disabled, and unemployed members. Some employers may even reimburse you for your professional memberships. It doesn't hurt to ask.

Tell me one more time why I should join and get active in my professional associations. In short, active membership is the best way to stay on the cutting edge of knowledge and information about your specialty and profession. It also provides a forum for sharing ideas and information, and is a wonderful way to support and celebrate the nursing profession. You can learn and develop your special interests and talents. It's a great way to meet nurses from other facilities and specialties, gain access to industry leaders, and find role models and mentors. In the end, membership gives you a competitive edge.

If you don't belong to professional associations, you become an observer with an obstructed view of your profession, rather than an active participant. By becoming involved, you become part of the solution, rather than part of the problem.

You can find out more about professional associations in nursing by going online to www.aacn.nche.edu/Education/reflist.htm or to www. nursingworld.org and clicking on Constituent Member Associations.

If you're still not ready to join for some reason, go to a local meeting as a guest. I don't know of any professional association that doesn't welcome guests to their meetings. This way, you can check out the programs and the people first before making a decision to join. You can also attend conferences and conventions as a nonmember. It's also okay to join now and ease your way in slowly. Even if you only get out to a few meetings the first year, that's progress!

Work On Your Education

Ongoing education is a necessary part of career development. So much changes in our daily lives and nursing practice that you have to incorporate learning into your everyday routine. Education is not just about career advancement — it's about staying involved and active. If you're not learning, you're stagnating.

Education can be formal or informal. Let's discuss the formal bit first. Many nurses cringe at the thought of returning to school in any capacity. But unless you already have an advanced degree, formal education should be in your plans. If you want to be taken seriously in nursing, you need essential educational credentials. More important, formal education will enrich your life in ways you can't imagine.

A bachelor's degree has become a minimum standard for any professional today. For those who attended a diploma or associate degree program, start making plans to return to school for a bachelor's degree. Don't think about it, just do it. And once you have a bachelor's degree, start thinking about graduate school. Some programs will allow you to work on your bachelor's and master's degrees simultaneously.

I often hear nurses say, "I'm going to retire in a few years," or, "I don't want to get into management, so why should I go back to school?" Formal education will support your career in many direct and indirect ways. However, the personal benefits far outweigh any potential career benefits. Education is a gift you give yourself. It keeps you young and makes you feel alive. It keeps your mind active. Education helps you to see the world in an expanded way with a better understanding of yourself and the world around you. It allows you to participate in a grander way. So, go back to school for yourself first and your career second. Even if they are planning to retire soon or stay in their current positions, many nurses end up shifting their plans unexpectedly by choice or by circumstances. You never know when and how a degree will come in handy.

Usual Objections to More Schooling

When enrolling in school, don't think about how old you'll be when you graduate. That's sure to sabotage your plans. Just get started, keep moving forward, and eventually you'll get to the end. And you'll want to avoid the following objections and self-imposed barriers to continuing your formal education:

I'm not smart enough. That's the way a lot of us feel, but every nurse is intelligent. How do I know that? Any licensed nurse has gotten through nursing school and passed a rigorous licensing exam. Plus, nurses handle complex care every day. If you made it this far as a nurse, you can definitely go the distance in higher education. It may not be easy, but you'll amaze yourself when you stretch your mental capacity and see just how much you are capable of learning and mastering. In fact, formal education, once completed, will validate your intelligence.

I don't have the time. Most of us have little free time, but we do have the ability to set aside time for things that are important to us. You may have to give up some volunteer work, delegate household chores, or pay someone to mow your grass or run some errands. There are all sorts of creative solutions to time challenges. Keep in mind that it's a temporary situation. You'll be in school for a limited amount of time.

· ·

My Personal Educational Journey

I was never much of a student. I scraped by during my basic education years. I just managed to struggle through a diploma in nursing program. The day I graduated, I was a happy camper, believing I would never have to sit in a classroom again.

Years later, as I contemplated what to do with the rest of my life and career, I began to think that beefing up my credentials would probably be a smart thing to do. I wasn't interested in earning a degree in nursing, so I enrolled in a bachelor of science in a healthcare management program.

I was scared to death to go back to school. Wouldn't everyone be younger and smarter than me? I wondered how long I could fool my professors into thinking I actually had something of value to contribute. When I finally got started, I was amazed that my fellow students were primarily my age, also working and taking care of a family. We were all in the same boat. Everyone supported and helped one another.

I decided to get started and plow ahead. I couldn't think about how long it would take me, because that thought was overwhelming to me. I had to focus on taking one step at a time. I knew if I kept moving forward, someday I'd be finished. When I did finally graduate several years later, I had a great sense of accomplishment. I felt more confident, more whole, and better prepared to face the world. You can't appreciate what higher education will do for you until you have it. It does change you for the better, whether you immediately recognize it or not.

Years later, I began to contemplate graduate school. I sat on the fence for years, not sure what degree I wanted to pursue. When I finally found the pro-

· ·

I don't have the money. Few of us have much disposable income, but money can be found for education. More money is available than most people realize and with a little time and effort, you can finance all or part of your schooling. Start by contacting the financial aid office at any school you plan to attend to locate scholarships, grants, and student loans. Professional associations, corporations, and other outside agencies and organizations offer funding. Some groups will even give you money for living expenses. You'll find many excellent books in the public library that list various scholarships and offer tips about how to go after them. There is an

gram I wanted to enroll in, a master's degree in corporate and public communication, I impulsively enrolled before I had much time to think about it and change my mind. I knew I was making a long-term commitment, but the way I looked at it, five years would pass whether I was in school or not. At the end of those years, I could either have a graduate degree, or I could still be thinking about it. I'm glad I bit the bullet and went for it.

Remember the movie *The Wizard of Oz?* The scarecrow always felt inadequate because he didn't think he had a brain. At the end of the movie, the wizard tells him that the only difference between him and great scholars is a diploma, which he hands the scarecrow. The scarecrow, with diploma in hand, immediately begins to think great thoughts, solve complex equations, and articulate beautifully. The diploma itself didn't make the scarecrow smart. Rather, it validated something in him that allowed him to realize his full potential. That's what my graduate degree, and accompanying diploma, did for me. It validated my mental competence, and it was an empowering and emotional experience.

While in graduate school, great opportunities came my way. For example, I was asked to write a research-based article for a nursing magazine and was approached about submitting a proposal to do some consulting for a large corporation. If I had not recently learned how to do both of those things in class, I might have turned my back on those and other opportunities, feeling ill-prepared to do so. Graduate school seemed to be preparing me for bigger and better challenges every step of the way. I always said that my formal education was the wave that was propelling me into the future. When I was finishing graduate school, people would ask me, "What are you going to do with your degree?" I'd tell them, "It's not what I'm going to do with that degree, but what that degree has already done for me." It has already made a difference in my life.

art and a science to successfully financing your education. Also, many employers offer tuition reimbursement, so find out what's available where you work. Funding should never be an obstacle to going back to school.

I'm too old to go back to school. If you really believe that age is an obstacle to learning, you might as well throw in the towel on life. Age is a state of mind. If you want to remain young at heart and stay fully engaged in life, get more education. You're never too old to go back to school. And if you're feeling old, school may be just the thing to rejuvenate you.

I didn't enjoy my undergraduate experience, and I don't want to repeat it. You're not alone. Undergraduate school was a struggle for many of us. Part of that challenge is the volume of credits required to graduate and a diverse core curriculum of demanding subjects. Although I struggled through some classes, they expanded my world and enriched my life in some way. However, graduate school is different. Your curriculum is more focused. Your projects and papers can be tailored to your areas of interest within your major. You have more flexibility and freedom in these studies.

FAQs About Continued Schooling

Besides objections, nurses often express common concerns and questions in making choices about continuing their formal education. Here are a few frequently asked questions.

Do I need to get my degrees in nursing? Earning an undergraduate or graduate nursing degree is a natural choice for some, but not for others. If teaching nursing or getting a doctorate in nursing is in your future, then a degree in nursing is the way to go. Otherwise, you've got other choices.

Which degree will give me the best job prospects and the highest earning potential? No one degree is right for any situation. If you interview hospital, healthcare, and nursing administrators and managers, you'll discover that they have degrees in different majors. If you talk with nursing professors, you'll find that although they all have graduate degrees in nursing, the focuses of their degrees may be very different. If you talk to successful nurses, you'll discover that some have degrees in nursing and others in diverse majors, such as healthcare administration, business, education, communication, public health, and even journalism.

ADN or BSN?

The nursing community has been engaged in much discussion about eventually making the BSN a standard for entry to practice. Discussion has also ensued about requiring future graduates of diploma and associate degree programs to obtain a BSN within a certain number of years after graduation (This will not affect those currently licensed). And while both of these concepts are still in the discussion phase, they underscore the fact that the BSN degree may hold more weight, especially in the clinical setting, in years to come. This is something to consider when choosing a major.

Any college degree will never guarantee career success. That is largely up to you. Which degree you pursue is an individual choice based on your career goals and interests. Your best bet is to choose a course of study that interests and excites you and then find a way to make it work for you. We'll talk more about the decision-making process and clarifying career goals in Chapter 3.

Are online programs as good as traditional programs? If an online program is appropriately accredited, it shares the same legitimacy as a traditional one. Since online degrees are so prevalent today, even at the doctoral level, they are widely accepted. Both distance learning and traditional classroom learning have their advantages and disadvantages. Fully explore both options before choosing the one that's right for you. It is helpful and advisable to talk to students who have completed both online and traditional classroom-based programs before deciding what's right for you. Every student has different needs and interests

Where can I find more information about schools, majors, and accreditation status? A few sources of information include the National League for Nursing (www.nln.org), American Academy of Colleges of Nursing (www.aacn.nche.edu), the *College Blue Book* found in the reference section of the library, and *Peterson's Graduate Schools in the U.S.* and other Peterson's guides (www.petersons.com).

Ongoing Education and Training

In addition to formal education, there are many other opportunities to keep your brain sharp. Here are just a few.

Participate in CE. You may live in a state that requires CE in the form of a certain number of contact hours for license renewal. Aside from that, CE should be a way of life for a professional. Opportunities abound for sanctioned nursing CE through seminars and classes, print publications, and online sources. But there are plenty of other avenues for ongoing learning, too.

See what's offered through your local adult school programs. Many colleges and universities offer noncredit courses and certificate programs in various subjects. Don't restrict your learning to clinical topics. Work on improving your skills in communication, writing, public speaking, and anything else that interests you or can enhance your knowledge, skill set, or expertise.

Work on your computer skills. Computers are an integral part of our life and work. If you don't already have good computer skills, take steps to get up to speed or you'll be left behind. Although computers are still intimidating to some, once you master the basics, your confidence level will soar. You'll also be more marketable.

Developing good computer skills includes becoming familiar with the Internet and knowing how to use it. Once you do, you'll have instant access to endless information and resources and be able to communicate with friends and colleagues around the world. If you're not yet hooked up to the Internet at home, you're missing out on so much. Get connected now.

Adult schools and community colleges have classes for computer users from beginner to advanced levels. Many public libraries offer free courses about how to use computers and the Internet. If you prefer to learn in the privacy of your own home, hire a computer tutor or ask your children or grandchildren to teach you. Experienced friends and family members can be a great help and are usually happy to assist.

Get to the library. Your public library is a vast source of almost totally free information. You can find books and multimedia products that address any subject under the sun. Whether you want to learn about Medicare regulations, how to write an article for publication, or acquire management skills, you'll find plentiful resources in the library. Be sure to check out the books on tape and educational videos, too.

College and healthcare facility libraries are great resources. With very few exceptions, both allow the general pubic to use their facilities. Of course, you might not be able to take any books out if you're not a student, employee, or alumnus there, but you can read, research, and take notes as needed. If you use the library of a university that offers degrees in nursing, you'll likely find a vast number of nursing and healthcare journals in their periodicals section.

Don't hesitate to ask the librarian or research assistant to help you find what you're looking for, either online or on the shelves. That's what they're there for and they're generally willing to help you.

Get certified in your specialty. If you have a few years of experience in a particular specialty and think you might continue to work in that area, look into getting certified. Certification based on experience and education is a measure of competency and a standard of excellence. It gives you higher standards to strive for in your practice and will, in many cases, make you more marketable.

However, do not confuse experience-based certification — the type that requires a certain number of hours/years worked in the specialty to qualify — with the type you can get after taking a one-day or one-week course with no previous experience in that field. Sanctioned certification is usually

Get Over It and On with It

"I was very intimidated about using computers, but knew I needed to learn. I heard that a local Girl Scouts chapter was offering computer classes for a minimal fee, so I signed up. The class was small and very helpful. We were all adults attending in the evening. It helped me get over my fears and learn the basics," Agnes, a middle-aged nurse with technophobia.

offered by professional associations and accrediting bodies, as opposed to those offered by other parties. Certification is only meaningful and valuable if it is based on experience and knowledge. The exception would be a "skills" certification that you receive after taking a course for something like IV administration, CPR, or specialized computer skills.

Get a grip on the big picture. Nurses have a tendency to focus solely on their current specialty. That's fine, but you have got to broaden your knowledge base of the bigger issues that affect nursing and healthcare, as well as the world around you. How can you effectively plan your career and know what specialties will be hot and growing if you are not aware of the trends and issues that will shape future healthcare and nursing?

Find out what healthcare economists are predicting for the next five to ten years. Learn about the concept of universal healthcare and its possible effects on the workplace. Everyone in healthcare is talking about mandated staffing ratios. Are you fully aware of the pros and cons? Get the facts so you have an informed opinion.

Where can you find all this information? It's just a few computer clicks away. Use the Internet to search for related topics, using key phrases such as "healthcare industry forecasts" and "nursing career trends." Spend some time in the library and online reading healthcare and nursing news magazines, such as *Nursing Spectrum* and *NurseWeek, Nursing Economic$,* and *Modern Healthcare.* Challenge your brain and expand your perspective with mainstream newspapers and news magazines as well.

Casting a Wide Network

Networking is one of the most important activities you can do for personal and professional success. It's all about connections. It's about meeting new people and developing relationships as well as staying in touch with those you already know. Think of your network as a support team, an information pipeline, a safety net, and a personal think tank of sorts. Networking allows you to tap into the collective wisdom, experience, and connections of those in your "virtual community." Because we live in a communication age, almost anyone in the universe can become part of that community.

While some people think of networking as a one-way situation where someone of importance pulls strings for you, it is actually a reciprocal process of giving and getting information and support. Networking is an interactive two-way street. Under the best circumstances, it is mutually beneficial.

Networking is misunderstood and highly underused by nurses. Why are we so reluctant to develop a network? Maybe because of the confidential nature of the work we do. We've become so accustomed to staying quiet that we're often reluctant to talk to others. Some of us are rusty with our socialization skills. Others may feel competitive and insecure, believing it's better to tough it out on their own, rather than giving and receiving help and support.

Some nurses think that everyday networking is superficial and pointless. I recently heard a nurse say, "I can't see the purpose of schmoozing just for schmoozing's sake." Schmoozing is a slang term for networking, and as such, it always has a purpose, even if only to stay connected to people you already know or to meet new people. One of the very exciting things about networking is that you never know who you're going to meet or run into.

By effectively developing and using a network, you can —

- Achieve your goals more quickly
- Stay completely up-to-date on issues and information
- Be more effective in your current job
- Share ideas and information
- Increase your chances of getting a promotion or breaking into a particular specialty
- Get additional and secondary contacts to expand your network
- Find out about a company, a specific job, or a specialty
- Get introductions to industry leaders, decision makers, and other influential people
- Discover hidden jobs that exist in a company but are not publicly advertised
- Develop a "virtual" support system that goes where you go

Where can you network? Out of all the different ways to network, face-to-face networking is the most effective. When you meet someone in person, you get a face to go with the name and have the opportunity to share a handshake and make eye contact. You get a sense of who the person is and vice versa. In-person encounters are generally more productive and memorable. Likewise, periodically seeing the people you know is always better than merely keeping in touch through other distant means. There is greater opportunity for interaction and communication. Here are some good places for face-to-face networking.

Professional association meetings: I've already mentioned the benefits of being active in professional associations, but your network should expand beyond nursing and even beyond healthcare. Consider attending an occasional chamber of commerce meeting, associations of professional business people, and other healthcare professions' meetings. You don't need to be a member of an organization or even work in a particular field to attend a few meetings as a guest.

Ask a few colleagues what organizations they belong to and ask to tag along to a meeting. It's always easier to go with someone you know, especially the first time. However, you have to make a point to talk to at least one new person while you're there, or you defeat the purpose of going.

Job fairs: Contrary to popular belief, job fairs are not just for job seekers. They're a great place to meet people and stay in touch with those you already know. In addition to the array of prospective employers exhibiting, schools of higher learning are usually represented as well, along with an occasional publisher, medical product company, and other vendors. An added benefit is sometimes a wide array of CE programs offered on such diverse subjects as stress management, bioterrorism, public speaking skills, and clinical topics.

Some job fairs are for nursing, some are for the healthcare industry in general, and others are for a specific industry, such as the pharmaceutical industry. Other job fairs are general in nature and include healthcare as well as nonhealthcare companies. You never know who you'll meet at these events, what companies will be represented, and what opportunities will be available. Even if you're content working where you are, you should always be exploring your options. Besides, the best time to look for your next job is while you're happily employed.

If you're worried someone will see you there and tell your boss who may, in turn, think that you're looking for another job, solve that problem by telling your boss beforehand that you're going. You might say you're contemplating going back to school and want to talk to the educational exhibitors who will be there. You can also say you want to attend the CE programs.

Conventions: You don't have to be a member of an organization to attend its convention. Many conventions offer special registration options for one day versus the entire event. I once attended a medical convention with a friend who is a physician. I had a blast. I attended a workshop on healthcare reimbursement issues and discovered I knew more about the subject than most of the physicians in the audience. I also attended a workshop there on dressing well for my body type and coloring. I found it very helpful.

Alumni events: Alumni have an immediate camaraderie with one another and a special bond, regardless of their year of graduation or their major. And since many alumni have great connections and influence, it pays to stay in touch. Use your alumnus status as a connection. Don't hesitate to mention it in conversation or in correspondence. It immediately builds trust. You might, for example, find out that a director of nursing or chief executive officer (CEO) of a particular healthcare system is a fellow graduate of your school.

Seminars and educational programs: When you attend educational activities, you can network with the speakers, the attendees, and those running the event. But don't ignore others in the vicinity. Whenever I attend any type of meeting or event at a hotel or conference center, I always scan the schedule to see who else is meeting there. I have often stopped in on another meeting to meet the event organizers or speakers during their breaks. The opportunities are endless when you get yourself out there.

Asking for Help

Years ago, when I was hired as director of DRG (diagnostic-related groups) Services, I was told that I'd eventually be responsible for the quality improvement (QI) department. I had no experience in that specialty whatsoever. When the time came for me to organize that department, I got on the telephone and called several area hospitals and asked to speak with their director of QI. I introduced myself and asked for their help. I asked what I should do first, what associations I should join, what key issues I needed to know about, and if they could send me a copy of their policy and procedure manual. Everyone was gracious and eager to help. We all stayed in touch after that and shared information and resources. We created a local network that was mutually supportive and beneficial.

"A smart man knows everything; a shrewd man, everyone."

Anonymous

Community activities: Get out to the occasional political rally, school board meeting, church social, or school fair. Even block parties provide great networking opportunities. You'll be amazed at the information you'll gather and the connections you'll make just by letting people in your circle, even casual acquaintances, know more about yourself and your goals, and finding out more about them. Find a way to mention in conversation that you're job hunting, starting a business, or interested in breaking into a particular specialty or working for a particular company or agency. That type of self-revelation can help to uncover hidden resources in your own backyard.

Anywhere there are people: Once you develop a networking mindset and become accustomed to talking to people, you'll be amazed at the interesting people you'll meet and run into virtually anywhere. I have met celebrities, CEOs, famous authors, and many interesting nurses and others on trains, planes, shuttle buses, and in the beauty parlor!

How to find out about meetings and conferences: To stay current with meetings and other related activities, view event calendars in nursing magazines and websites. Check out the community events calendar in your local newspaper. Ask colleagues to keep you informed of upcoming meetings and conferences and to pass on brochures to you. You can also contact various organizations and ask to be put on their mailing lists.

Other ways to stay in touch: The Internet is a great networking tool. Join listservs, participate in bulletin boards, and join in on the occasional live chat. These are all forums for letting off steam, sharing information and ideas, garnering support, and keeping up with what's happening. You can find these forums on professional association, general nursing, and career websites. Some general and specialty listservs exist independently. Find a list of those by doing an Internet search for "nursing listservs" and "nursing discussion forums."

E-mail is a great way to stay in touch with people and even to make a preliminary contact with someone before calling them. While e-mail is not an appropriate form of communication in every situation, it is a fast, easy way to stay in touch. It can also serve as an introduction or provide easy access to influential people. You can even reach the president of the U.S. via e-mail!

In many cases, there's nothing like picking up the telephone and actually talking to someone. In fact, if you are accustomed to e-mailing someone all the time, be sure to occasionally speak with him or her by phone. It's more personal and interactive. And some people find it easier to speak by phone than to have to type a response through e-mail.

Of course there's always the U.S. Postal Service (USPS). Traditional mail, also known as "snail mail" in computer lingo, is a great way to stay in touch

Staying in Touch Online

An e-mail list, or listserv, is a type of virtual community made up of people with common interests. Once you subscribe to a list, usually at no cost, messages are delivered directly into your personal e-mail account. Only members of that list are privy to the messages, or "posts." You can read the posts that interest you based on the subject line, respond to the group if you wish, ask a question, start your own discussion, or just observe without active participation, which is known as "lurking." Some examples of a listserv focus include psychiatric nursing, telehealth, case management, and student nurses. Some lists are even related to particular nursing theorists and nursing history. Other listservs are general in nature and any nursing-related topic is fair game. Some lists are relatively inactive and others are very busy, generating multiple posts per day.

A bulletin board, message board, or online discussion forum exists in cyberspace and anyone can view the board by going to the appropriate web address. If you wish to participate by posting a comment or question or responding to another post, you'll usually be asked to log in on the site each time you wish to participate. However, generally anyone can read and search the forums without having to log in. Messages are categorized by specific discussion topics, or "threads." You can usually "search" these forums to find out what has already been said on a particular topic.

A live chat is a cyber conversation that takes place in real time. Some live chats are hosted by experts and have a specific theme or topic. Others simply are "open" during certain hours of certain days, and anyone can sign on and either participate or lurk. Obviously, you can only chat with those who happen to be online at the same time as you. Some chats get very lively, and it is challenging to keep up. Others are slower paced and more manageable. Try signing on sometime to get a feel for what goes on and how it works.

through the use of greeting cards or an occasional handwritten note to say "Thanks" or "Congratulations." In this electronic age, people appreciate the personal, low-tech forms of communication.

Usual Objections to Networking

Just as a litany of excuses is used as justification for not joining organizations or continuing education, networking detractors have raised their own unworthy objections.

I don't have time to network. We all have schedules that seem maxed out. We all feel tired and overwhelmed. The amazing thing is that networking can energize you. The connections you make, the interesting people you meet, the support and energy you gather, and the ideas and information you pick up through networking stimulate you. Networking also lessens your feelings of being alone, helping you feel upbeat and hopeful with a sense of being part of a greater whole.

I can't get out of the house. Maybe your work schedule or childcare issues prevent you from attending formal networking events. Try to make arrangements beforehand to get the time off or have someone help you out at home. Even if you can't get out, formal events are not the only place to network. We all come in contact with people at work, at the grocery store, through our children's school, and through social activities. Opportunities exist everywhere. Remember, networking is not confined to nursing and healthcare circles. Additionally, you always have the Internet, telephone, and USPS.

I'm too shy and nervous. There are always those who seem to be able to work a room like a pro, but they have usually learned and practiced their networking skills out of necessity or desire. The truth is, most people consider themselves shy networkers. If you don't get out much, as many nurses do not, your socialization skills get rusty. Of course, some of us may not have been very good at it to begin with.

Many people are uncomfortable socializing because they have trouble remembering people's names. They may be uncomfortable making conversation, or they may not know how to break the ice with strangers. These are skills that can be learned and mastered with a little know-how and practice.

Networking is a pervasive theme throughout this book because it's very important. This section serves merely as an introduction to the whys and wheres of networking. The how-tos and other important uses for networking will be discussed in more depth in subsequent chapters.

Moving Forward, Where Do I Go From Here?

While a handful of nurses have a clear idea of where they want to be five years from now, most do not. I frequently hear nurses say, "I don't know what I want to be when I grow up," and these are not necessarily young nurses. Most of us just keep doing what we've been doing without giving much thought about, or doing much planning for our future. It's so easy to get stuck in a rut. That's when what you do ceases to become a career and becomes just a job.

Many people are under the mistaken belief that if they don't know what they want to do, they can't move forward until they make that decision. On the contrary, you have to start moving forward, creating some momentum in your professional life, to discover what you're good at, where your special talents and interests lie, and where the opportunities are. Indecision won't solve anything. It will only magnify self-doubt and anxiety.

While some nurses do exactly the same thing for years on end, others haphazardly hop around from job to job on an eternal quest to find their niche. They often do this, unfortunately, without considering what they enjoy doing, what they're good at, or what their ideal work environment might be. When they don't take time to explore their own wants and needs and get in tune with their strengths and assets, they waste a lot of time looking for career satisfaction in a place of employment, rather than looking for that satisfaction within themselves. Instead, they should think about their own interests and then look for a position that supports those interests, rather than taking any job that comes along hoping they'll discover it will suit them.

All About You

As nurses, we are versatile and multitalented, but we are notorious for underestimating our own value and capabilities. We are good at so many different things. These abilities are so second nature to us that we may not see them as assets. We are so accustomed to doing whatever comes our way that we lose sight of how creative, skillful, and knowledgeable we are.

So what exactly are we so good at? We are master multitaskers. We juggle so many balls at one time, and we're not juggling light-weight Styrofoam balls either; it's more like keeping a chain saw, a flaming torch, a live chicken, and a fragile piece of china in the air. I used to tell prospective employers that for every year I worked in the hospital, I got two years worth of experience. I was making a point about the work, responsibilities, and new knowledge I acquired on an ongoing basis, as well as the actions I had to initiate in the drama of a typical nurse's day.

Nurses are organized, detail oriented, and acutely aware of their surroundings. We think on our feet, making quick decisions and managing complex projects. We're excellent problem solvers and are totally customer-service oriented. Nurses possess excellent communication skills. We regularly translate complex material into terms that can be understood by the variety of people with whom we interact. We often adjust our language and our style of speaking from moment to moment without conscious thought, communicating with an array of people, from those with big egos to those under extreme stress. And we have to do this with a culturally diverse population.

Here is a partial list of strengths and assets of the average nurse:

Skills	Attributes
Analyzing	Adaptable
Communicating effectively	Creative
Counseling/Coaching	Dependable
Decision making	Detail oriented
Organizing	Flexible
Planning	Hard working
Presenting/Speaking	Innovative
Problem solving	People oriented
Developing programs	Reliable

Writing reports	Resourceful
Researching	Responsible
Selling (yes, selling!)	Has a sense of humor
Supervising/Managing	Functions as a team player
Teaching/Training	Thinks on his or her feet
Team leading	Works independently
Managing time	Works well under pressure

Transferable Skills

In addition to the talents and abilities that nurses use every day in traditional healthcare settings, they also possess many skills that can be transferred to other areas of practice. For example, nurses are natural teachers. We instruct all the time without thinking about it. And we are engaged in public speaking, which is nothing more than teaching on a grander scale.

Nurses are natural salespeople, too. We have to "sell" constantly in the clinical setting. Every time you have to convince a patient to adhere to a regimen or follow up on a test, you are selling. An even harder sell is when you have to convince a member of the healthcare team that something is a good idea when they don't see it that way. You are pointing out the benefits to the buyer, overcoming objections, and closing the sale. We do that everyday in nursing. These skills are easily transferable to product, pharmaceutical, and service sales.

Nurses also possess a great body of knowledge and experience that is very valuable and transferable to many settings including legal nurse consulting, research, writing, and consulting. Remember when I was offered the position of center manager at the weight control center and was convinced I couldn't do it? I quickly learned that my nursing instincts, assessment skills, decision-making capabilities, brains, and prior experience had actually prepared me well for the business world. But of course, at the time, I still had that "just a nurse" mentality.

Self-Assessment

A fundamental first step in developing a career plan is to do an honest self-assessment. This is not something you can develop in an hour. You need some time to think about it, reflect on past experiences, and talk with those who know you well.

Exercise

Get a notebook, legal pad, a journal, or sit at your computer. Write down or type the following questions. Then take some time to ponder the answers and write down your thoughts. It may take you a month or more to compile an accurate profile. It is important to write these things down and not just think about them. Why? Because putting pen to paper or fingers to keyboard takes something from the abstract and makes it concrete. It helps to clarify your thoughts and desires. It gives you a visual reference to read, re-read, and re-write.

Question #1: What do I enjoy doing?

Does the challenge of hands-on care make your heart beat faster? Do you love teaching and working with students and new hires? Is writing something you have a passion for? Are you interested more in the big picture of things — project management, budget development, staffing studies? Does public policy excite you? Write down anything that makes you feel excited or challenged, that feeds your creative side, or that gives you satisfaction. It doesn't matter if you think you can make a living at it, or if you think it is practical for you or even if you think you're "any good" at it. Just write it down. Many of us never take the time to think about what we really enjoy doing, yet that should be at the heart of everything we do in our career.

Years ago, I received a call from a distraught nurse. She had just gone on an interview for a position she really wanted and was turned down for the job. She felt lost and deflated and was looking for guidance. She told me she had been an oncology nurse for 15 years and had applied for a position to do some counseling for a new program being started by a pharmaceutical company. The prospective employer had seen her résumé and called her in for an interview. I asked her how the interview went, and she said she thought it went well.

This nurse proceeded to tell me that she made it clear to the interviewer that she didn't have any counseling experience. She further advised them that she was willing to learn and take any courses they wanted to send her to, but again emphasized she didn't have any experience. In reality, this nurse had 15 years of counseling experience as an oncology nurse. She just didn't see it. Instead, she went to great lengths to talk her way out of a job. This is one very unfortunate example of how nurses are often unable to identify innate skills and abilities and transfer them to other areas of practice.

If you're still not sure what you enjoy, become more self-aware in your everyday work. What parts of your job do you enjoy the most and the least? Think about things you've done in the past that have given you satisfaction, enjoyment. And by the way, it doesn't have to be strictly related to nursing and healthcare. Many a nurse has combined his or her nursing career with a seemingly unrelated interest such as flying, sports, music, or the outdoors.

Question #2: What am I good at?

Each of us has special talents and abilities. Certain things come easy to us or seem to be natural. Others admire us for certain traits and often seek our advice or help on related issues. Is there something people have complimented you on or told you you're good at, whether you agree with them or not?

If you're not sure what you do well, or even if you think you are, ask a few people who know you well what they see as your strong points. You may be pleasantly surprised by the response you get and discover something positive about yourself. Often our strong points are so much a part of who we are, we do not necessarily see them as such. In other words, we take them for granted.

Question #3: What am I interested in?

Maybe you've been curious to learn more about computers and how they work in healthcare. Perhaps you're intrigued by a different specialty or type of employer. Have you always thought you'd like to learn more about holistic healing and wellness? Maybe the law has always fascinated you, and you've wondered if that field might be right for you. Write down everything you can think of, putting those that intrigue you most at the top.

Many nurses have told me they have absolutely no idea what they want to do or what they're interested in. Yet, when pressed, there is often something hovering just below the surface. I once spoke with a nurse who was frantically trying to change her career, but couldn't identify any special interests. I took the conversation in another direction and she revealed that she loved to write and had always wanted to pursue that. When I pointed out that she had just revealed something she actually did have a strong interest in, she snapped, "Nobody makes any money at that." In reality, there are many nurses making a part- or full-time living by writing. However, many of us resist our own thoughts and desires because of fears, preconceived notions about ourselves and other things, and expectations we, our family, and our friends have of us. Everyone dreams about something, whether they want to admit it or not. Sometimes the dream is so well hidden and buried so deep that we even forget it exists.

Question #4: What transferable skills do I have?

Ask yourself, "What have I done? What are my experiences?" Transferable skills are those things you have experience with that can be used in alternate settings or in alternative ways. Nurses have a tendency to focus solely on their clinical skills. However, as previously mentioned, nurses are excellent at many other things. Focus on any business or managerial experience you've had such as working on schedules or budgets. Do you ever take a charge position or supervisory role on your unit, even if only occasionally? How about working with students or new hires? Have you developed an educational tool or fact sheet? Have you presented at grand rounds, presented in-services, been liaison to outside agencies?

Question #5: What areas do I need/want to improve in?

Maybe you need to get a new updated look in terms of your hairstyle and clothing. We all get in ruts with our appearance as well as our work. Perhaps your communication skills need some work. Maybe you need to expand your computer skills or advance your formal education. You might need to find some creative outlets or down time to create some balance and harmony in your life. Write down whatever you can think of. Focus on both professional and personal things since the two go hand in hand.

Question #6: What would my ideal work environment be like?

Think about the type of environment you'd like to work in and the parameters of your work life. For example, would you prefer a patient care area vs. a business setting vs. a home-based office? Would you prefer to be stationary or "on the road" sometimes? Would you prefer to work regular "business hours" or have flexible scheduling that might include weekends, holidays, shift work? Are you looking for 12 hour shifts, part-time work, or per diem?

"I often push myself to try new things in order to step out of my personal boundaries and to learn more about myself. It seems that most people don't understand their own strengths and weaknesses until they compare themselves to others or until they put themselves in a completely new and different situation. When I attend professional association meetings, get involved in a new project, or try my hand at something new, I realize my own good qualities and shortcomings more clearly."

Catherine

Finding Your Niche

Now that you've done your self-assessment, you still don't know what you want to be when you grow up, right? Again, that's normal for most of us. Many nurses get so hung up on finding what they believe is that one right job or specialty, the elusive niche that they forget to savor the process of getting there. You've probably heard the expression, "Success is a journey not a destination." That means you have to focus more on the process and be less focused on the outcome.

I'm always amazed when I hear a new graduate nervously say they haven't found their niche yet, when they've barely started their career. We put such pressure on ourselves to discover our place. Some of us think we'll have a revelation of sorts. In reality, that "niche" will likely change from time to time and will evolve as you move forward. As you read in Chapter 1, I tried on many hats before getting to where I am today. Have I reached my final career destination yet? I doubt it. I'm still a traveler.

In order to focus on the process, you need actions and activities that will lead you down a path of discovery about yourself, your opportunities, and the world around you. Keep in mind that you don't need to know exactly where you're headed or exactly what you want to do in order to get on with your life and career. However, by moving in a positive, forward direction, the right path will eventually reveal itself to you. In other words, you've got to move forward in faith.

Ideas, inspiration, and enlightenment come from the most unexpected sources and in the most unexpected ways and places. That's why it's important to initiate action and activity, or "create momentum," in your professional life. Here are ways to do just that.

1. Accumulate Experiences

There are lots of opportunities to stretch yourself in your professional life. By trying new things, you may find something you like or something you're good at. You'll also learn more about the bigger world of nursing and healthcare in general. These are all necessary steps to developing a career path.

- Offer to work on special projects at work. Try your hand at doing the schedule or department budget. Take a shot at being a preceptor to students and new graduates. Make yourself available to attend recruitment events or work at community health screening programs. Propose a department quality improvement project and offer to conduct the research and write up the report. These, and other related activities, will expose you to new things and force you to develop some new skills. By the way, I'm not suggesting you do these things out of a sense of loyalty to your employer, rather, I'm suggesting you do these things because of what's in it for you.

- Get on facility-wide committees. Find some interdisciplinary (interdepartmental) committees that interest you (such as a recruitment and retention, quality improvement, or safety committee) and volunteer to be a part of them. Getting on interdisciplinary committees is a good way to pick up new skills and experiences, expand your knowledge base, increase your influence, develop new relationships and learn something about yourself in the process.

2. Use Professional Associations as a Training Ground

Hopefully, I made a good case for why you should join and become active in professional associations in Chapter 2. But again, you never know how or where those experiences will work out for you.

Bob was an ICU nurse who was interested in learning new things. When his manager asked for a volunteer to sit on a new hospital-wide communication committee, Bob jumped at the chance. He asked how much time would be required and was told two to three hours per month, which he could do on work time. Bob said, "I thought it sounded interesting so I agreed to participate." The purpose of the committee was to evaluate how the various departments received and transmitted information. The committee would then be asked to make suggestions for improvement.

One of the recommendations that came from the committee was for the hospital to install a computerized patient charting system. Part of the proposal included creating a new full-time position to oversee the project installation, train all the employees, act as liaison to the hardware and software vendors, and be a troubleshooter. Once the proposal was approved, who do you think they offered that job to? Bob became the hospital's first Nursing Informatics Specialist and has never looked back.

Bob's experience can be summed up with a line from *A Hero in Every Heart* by H. Jackson Brown, Jr.: "Opportunity dances with those already on the dance floor."

When I launched my education business years ago, I started out by offering public seminars in my home state and later across the country. People would often ask me, "How did you ever learn to run seminars like that? How did you know what to do?" I responded, "Believe it or not, I learned while I was the Education Chair for a state professional association I belonged to years ago. As such, we ran an annual full day seminar. I had to negotiate with national speakers, contract with hotels, apply for continuing education credits, work with a graphic designer and printer to develop a brochure, market the program, and coordinate all onsite activities the day of the event." In that position, I also had to coordinate the association's exhibit booth at state conventions, something else that came in handy as a business owner.

Did I envision myself someday running my own seminars back then? The thought had never occurred to me. But Benjamin Disraeli once said, "The secret to being successful is to prepare for life's opportunities before they present themselves." So how can you prepare for something that hasn't happened yet? When any opportunity presents itself, consider it and think about what you might be able to learn rather than being so quick to say "no."

3. Showcase Your Special Talents and Interests

If you like to write, volunteer to work on the employee newsletter or develop some patient education materials. If you love to teach and speak, volunteer to present at grand rounds, do department in-services, or provide some community education. If technology is your cup of tea, offer to create a database for scheduling or quality improvement data. Show the world what you're capable of doing and develop your special talents at the same time.

Patti Rager, RN, is former president and publisher of Nursing Spectrum (now known as Gannett Healthcare Group), a communications company that publishes 13 regional *Nursing Spectrum* and *NurseWeek* magazines, reaching more than a million registered nurses and nursing students. Early in her nursing career, Patti took the initiative to develop her love of writing.

"I started newsletters for the nursing department and the community as a sideline in two consecutive hospital positions I held. After I completed my MBA, I took courses in a magazine certificate program. I was then recruited to launch the *Nursing Spectrum* magazine in Washington, DC. Little did I know that I had been 'practicing' to later become president and publisher of Nursing Spectrum! You never know what nurses will end up doing."

4. Use Volunteering as a Career Management Tool

Many people think of volunteering as something charitable you do to help others. Although that may be true, there are also many benefits to the volunteer. If you'd like to get some teaching experience, doing that as a volunteer for a social service organization like the American Red Cross or American Heart Association is a smart thing to do. Would you like experience organizing public events or using information technology? Volunteering your services to a clinic or local public health agency is a great way to get it. Volunteer experience is no less valid or meaningful than paid experience. It's wonderful to volunteer for altruistic reasons, but always look for the opportunities and consider the potential for personal growth in any situation.

5. Explore Career Options

The majority of nurses are not aware of the broad scope of opportunities that are available to them both in and out of the hospital. Not only do most nurses lack knowledge about various options, but they often have inaccurate, preconceived notions about certain specialties and positions based on outdated or incorrect information.

Even if you're happy in your current specialty, it's important to know what options are out there. Knowing you have options lessens your anxiety about the future. Each nurse should understand the full scope of what other nurses are doing.

Here are some ways to explore career options:

- Attend related seminars and workshops. Programs on specific specialties as well as general career option programs are offered by colleges, professional associations, communication companies, and private education companies.

- Get out to career fairs. These events generally offer presentations on specific career opportunities. Not only can you learn something, you can also talk with the speaker and others actually doing that thing. You can also discuss various types of career offerings with exhibitors.

- Get on the Internet. You'll find general nursing sites and related professional association websites with tons of information and resources about various specialties. You'll also find articles, guest lectures, live chats, etc. about various specialties. Use search phrases such as: "nursing career specialties," "nursing specialties," "career alternatives for nurses," or "nontraditional nursing specialties."

- Talk to other nurses you meet at meetings, in your workplace, or in other situations. Ask them to tell you about what they do.

- Attend some specialty professional association meetings as a guest. If you're considering working in the Operating Room (OR), for example, attend a local chapter meeting of the Association of periOperative Registered Nurses (AORN). Tag along with a friend or go by yourself.

6. Working with Counselors and Coaches

Sometimes a qualified professional can help you in your journey. Such a person can serve as an objective third party to help you identify your strengths, explore options, decide where you fit in, help you to effectively market yourself, and work on specific problems and challenges. They will not place you in a job as an employment agency or professional recruiter might, but they will assist you in that process.

Career counselors have a graduate degree in counseling and specialized education and training in career management. They must be licensed or certified. Many career counselors use standardized testing to identify personality traits and interests. These tests don't actually tell you what type of career or specialty you should be in, but rather tell you what fields people with similar traits are working in. Some career counselors can also help you develop a career plan and clarify career goals. They can be particularly helpful if you have specific personal or career challenges to deal with, such as a spotty work history, a disability, or a history of addiction.

Career coaches don't need to be licensed although some are certified by professional associations. They do some of the same things that a career counselor does, depending on their background and expertise. A coach might be characterized as a catalyst, a facilitator, or a "personal trainer" for career related issues. Like a career counselor, they can help you decide what's right for you and then help you get there. They can give you specific advice that will help you clarify goals, develop an action plan, and then hold you accountable to meet those goals.

Joan, a registered nurse and life/career coach, offers this definition of coaching: "The goal of coaching is to support and partner with you to move towards the goals that are meaningful to you, and away from what is holding you back. By focusing on the action steps you can take in the present, a coach helps you create the future you want."

If you seek the services of a coach or counselor for help with your career, consider one who is also a nurse. A nurse has unique insights into the special skills and abilities and psyche of nurses and should be familiar with the vast array of opportunities out there for nurses. Those outside of nursing sometimes hold a limited view of what we do and lack in-depth knowledge about related opportunities.

Where can you find these people? The best way to find a competent career professional is through word of mouth or personal referrals. In other words, ask around. You may be able to get a referral through a nursing or healthcare professional association as well as state and national associations of coaches and counselors. Some colleges, including your alma mater and other local schools, may offer free or nominal fee career services. You can also look in the yellow pages of your phone book and in magazine and newspaper classified ads under "services offered." Make sure the person you choose to work with has the expertise and skills you need and is someone you feel comfortable working with. Fees vary so be sure to ask about costs up front.

7. Mentors, Role Models, and Advisors

If there is someone you know whom you have a relationship with, work with, or admire from afar, consider having a brief conversation with them in person or by telephone to discuss career-related issues. Mentors, role models, and advisors take many forms. They might be someone doing something you aspire to do who can give you advice and support. They might be someone who is successful in their own right and can give insights and information about a particular industry or provide inspiration and encouragement to you. They might be someone who has overcome obstacles or adversity to get where they are and can motivate you to take your career to the next level. Read more about mentoring in Chapter 10.

Letting the Universe Work for You

You may have heard a cat owner say, "I didn't find the cat. The cat found me." Sometimes the same thing happens with a job. You may or may not be looking for a new position when an opportunity presents itself. It may be something you have never done before or never even considered doing. Yet, there are elements of the position and/or specialty that intrigue and attract you. If this happens to you, at the very least, gather more information, go on an interview if you have the opportunity, and take some time to think about what it might mean for you.

Be open to new ideas and opportunities. Sometimes a seemingly random event is the universe's way of lighting your path. One nurse recently said to me, "I've been unlucky in my career. I've been laid off four times in the last four years." I suggested that maybe fate was playing a hand and giving her a gentle boot out into the world of unconventional work options. When I suggested this, she admitted that she had always wanted to start her own nursing business but never had the courage to break out on her own. She suddenly saw her "misfortune" as an opportunity to move in a new direction. There is always more than one door.

Learn to listen to your inner voices and trust your instincts. We often resist that which pulls us or interests us. The philosopher Goethe said, "When you learn to trust yourself, you will know how to live." If you relax into your life, let down some of your defenses, and push away some of the brambles in your mind, you may see a path that was previously hidden from view. This internal "listening" and "knowing" sometimes requires spending quiet time away from the distractions of everyday life, including television and radio. The library, a park, a house of worship, a museum, or even a special room of your house can provide such space.

Challenges to Moving Forward

All this talk about stepping out of your comfort zone, creating momentum, expanding your horizons, and moving forward is probably making you a little nervous, right? That's normal. Following are some common obstacles to getting on with your career as well as some practical solutions for getting beyond them.

The Fear Factor

Fear is a powerful force in our lives. Too often, it keeps us from realizing our dreams, developing our full potential, and reaching self-actualization. Moving forward in your career involves making changes and trying new things, and that is scary stuff for most of us. As humans, we resist change and prefer to maintain the status quo, but no growth occurs without change. That doesn't mean you necessarily have to change jobs. It means you have to step out of your comfort zone and stretch yourself. Understand that whenever you're making changes or trying something new, fear is automatically part of the equation. If you didn't feel some degree of fear and anxiety than you wouldn't be challenging yourself. Even successful people are afraid of making changes, trying new things, and taking their careers to the next level. They have just learned to move forward in spite of that fear.

For some of us, fear becomes a self-imposed barrier that stands between us and our destiny. I once read a quote that said, "We are like prisoners in a cell where the door is open and the jailer is gone." That quote conjures up an image of the self-imposed imprisonment many of us put ourselves in. We never move forward in our careers because we fear failure and success, dread the unknown, are panicked by looking foolish, and are scared of not knowing what we're doing.

So how can you better cope with your fears?

- Acknowledge and accept them. Rather than letting fear become an obstacle, learn to bring it along with you as you move forward, knowing that it is part and parcel of stretching yourself. Think of it as growing pains. Mark Twain said, "Courage is resistance to fear, mastery of fear, not absence of fear."

- Look for support and encouragement from friends and family and like-minded individuals. I once heard someone say, "Sometimes you have to believe in someone else's belief in you until your own belief kicks in." If there's something you want to do, look to those who believe in you or others already doing that thing for support and guidance.

- Face your fears head on. Often, our fear of doing something is much worse than actually doing it. Remember, you only have to do something for the first time once. And, as already mentioned, nurses are highly intelligent individuals and quick learners. We're adaptable, flexible, and versatile. We're capable of much more than we give ourselves credit for.

- Get yourself pumped up and positive. Many fears are based on our feelings of inadequacy and self-doubt. And those feelings become magnified in the face of new challenges and transitions. Shift your focus by reading and listening to motivational materials. Write down positive things people have said about you. Make a list of your past accomplishments. We often think in terms of where we are now and where we still want to go. We forget about how far we've already come. When you focus on the positive, it becomes your reality. It also helps to put your fears into perspective.

Excuses, Excuses, Excuses

Instead of making commitments, many of us make excuses. We all have our favorite excuses that we're fond of using to convince ourselves why we can't do something or can't move forward in our lives. Excuses are simply self-made obstacles. Excuses usually take two forms; the, "I can't because," excuses and the, "I'm waiting for," excuses. Here are some typical excuses we use to create obstacles to moving forward.

"I can't because... I'm too old... I'm too young... I don't have the right experience... I'm not smart enough... I'm too fat... I've been in nursing too long... I've been out of nursing too long... my biorhythms are out of whack... I don't have a college degree... I don't have a high enough degree... I have too many advanced degrees." The list goes on and on. We have an incredible knack for taking our own circumstances and turning them into a convenient, yet unfounded, reason not to move forward. Here are some others.

"I'm waiting for... my kids to finish college... my kids to leave home... my spouse to leave home... my bank account to be bigger... circumstances to be ideal... my waist line to be smaller... hell to freeze over... a total eclipse of the sun." Many of these may never happen, but we cling steadfastly to them. And if one situation resolves itself, we can easily substitute another excuse to prolong our waiting, thus avoiding growth, to ad infinitum.

Believe me when I tell you that I have heard every excuse in the book at one time or another and even used some of them myself along the way. In reality, you can do anything you put your mind to. If you make something a priority in your life, you'll find a way to work it out. Every perceived obstacle can be overcome. And if you're waiting for circumstances to be what you envision as ideal in your life, you're setting yourself up for failure since so many other things can happen while you're waiting. You're making an assumption that everything will remain status quo in your life while you wait: your job, your health, your financial situation, your family structure, the economy, etc. In truth, there will never be a better time than now to move forward, even in some small way.

Indecision

Many of us sit on the fence for a good part of our career trying to decide which direction to move in. We avoid making decisions because we're afraid of living with the consequences of wrong decisions. But not making a decision is a decision in itself; it's a decision to keep things as they are, and there are consequences associated with that. The ability to make good career decisions is an important part of moving forward. We are more in control of our lives and careers than most of us want to admit. Anthony Robbins, the self-help guru, says, "I believe it's our decisions, not the conditions of our lives, that determine our destiny."

No career decisions are perfect nor are any wrong. There are only different paths to follow. You have to make career choices based on the best information available to you, where you are right now in your life and career, and where you might be headed. You should make those choices based on your interests, needs, instincts, and the options available to you.

Of course you can't always be certain of the outcome when you make a decision. You have to make your choice and move forward with faith.

Often, indecision is masking fear. We say, "I don't know what I want to do," when in reality the truth, or the action that would be required to make that truth a reality, is too frightening to think about. As mentioned above, some of us fear success as much as we fear failure and worry about how it will change our lives, others' perceptions of us, and our own view of the world. Of course, in some cases, we are simply overwhelmed with the sheer number of choices available and have trouble sorting through them all.

My Hero

Each of us has our heroes in nursing; someone we admire for their clinical skills, compassionate caring nature, level-headedness, or what they've done with their careers. One of my nursing heroes is a woman named Rosemary. We worked together years ago and stayed in touch over the years. She is one of the most competent and caring nurses I have ever known. Her intelligence, clear thinking, uncompromising values, nursing intuition, and commitment to her profession have always impressed me. I have learned much from her over the years. She is one of the quiet heroes of our profession.

I recently asked her why she became a nurse. I was interested to know what brought her to where she is today. Her answer shocked me. "I almost DIDN'T become a nurse after a high school guidance counselor told me I wasn't smart enough," she said. "I knew I wanted to be a nurse from the fifth or sixth grade. I had visited a Veteran's Administration hospital with a Girl Scout troop one Christmas holiday. There were a lot of very sick people there. All of my friends couldn't wait to leave, yet I wanted to stay. I was somehow drawn to the place, the patients. I almost felt as if I belonged there. I later wrote a school paper about the nursing profession and got an 'A' on it, and I didn't get too many A's back then!

"So when it became time to plot my future, I not only knew exactly what I wanted to do, but I even knew what nursing school I wanted to go to. When I relayed this to my guidance counselor, she uttered those words I will never forget 'You're not smart enough to be a nurse.' To add salt to the wound she added, 'Besides, you would never get accepted into that school.' I was devastated. I took her at her word and dropped my plans to follow my dream.

The good news is that good decision making, once you learn the appropriate steps, is something you get better at with practice.

How to facilitate the decision making process:

- Consider what you want and need based on self-assessment and your current level of career satisfaction and happiness. Is there something you need to change? Something you want to do? Something you'd like to try? Write down what is most important to you and what you're most interested in. Consider possible options and solutions.

Instead, I took an office job out of high school and was absolutely miserable.

"My mother knew how unhappy I was and in an effort to help, mentioned an LPN program being offered in our area to county residents. My guidance counselor's words rang in my head, and I thought to myself, 'But I'm not smart enough.' I decided to give it a shot anyway. As it turns out, I got a great education and happily worked as an LPN for 5 years. I then enrolled in a university program to become an RN/BSN. I was on a roll."

Over the years, Rosemary worked as a staff nurse in critical care, and was the charge nurse on a telemetry unit, manager in cardiac rehab, part of the staff education team, utilization review nurse, head nurse in oncology, and a member of the float pool. She eventually became a certified diabetic educator. Rosemary worked all of her RN career to that point in the same hospital. That is where I came to know her. I used to tease her that she should receive an award for having the most positions within the shortest amount of time at one place of employment. She had eight different positions in 18 years. She said, "I had so many interests and so many opportunities. I was always learning something new and was open to new challenges and experiences."

Years later, Rosemary decided to go to graduate school and become a nurse practitioner. She was ready to take her practice to the next level. After 5 years of blood, sweat, tears, and many personal sacrifices, Rosemary became a certified Adult Nurse Practitioner. Today, she has a collaborative arrangement with several physicians in a busy cardiology practice.

Rosemary's advice to others: "Be true to yourself. Don't ever let someone else tell you what you should or shouldn't do with your life. And don't let anyone else shatter your dreams. If you want to do something badly enough, there is always a way to do it. Go for it!"

- Gather more information. For example, if you're having difficulty deciding on a degree major, request some catalogs from nearby colleges and/or from online programs. This will allow you to review the coursework for various majors, the admission requirements, number of credits required, fees involved, etc. All of this is vital information in choosing a school and a major. You can also go the public library and browse through books in the reference section such as *The College Blue Book* which list schools and majors in volumes labeled "Healthcare," "Business," "Social Sciences," etc. You may discover a degree program you weren't aware of. Ask the librarian to help you find these and other related resources. The Internet can also be helpful.

If you're considering changing specialties, use the steps mentioned previously under "Explore Career Options." If you're considering starting a business, get to the pubic library or the Internet and see what's required to start a business in your state, including any special requirements for the specific type of business you're considering. You can't make an informed decision until you have all the facts.

- Talk to people in the know. Get in touch with people who have done something similar, who are working in a field you're considering, or have pursued a degree you're thinking about. They can give you a unique perspective and inside information that you may not have thought about. People have different opinions and experiences, so talk to several people and accept that you may have to sort through the advice and information to find what you need.

- Write about it. Writing can be very therapeutic and help to clarify your thoughts. Whether you put pen to paper or fingers to keyboard, the very act of writing down what's on your mind, including your questions and your dilemmas, can help you to work toward decisions and solutions.

- Talk it over with a friend or trusted colleague. When you have an important decision to make, talking it out can be very helpful. Saying things out loud gives you a different perspective than thinking about it or even writing about it. You can also get feedback and input from the person with whom you're speaking.

- Go with your gut. When all is said and done, only you can make a decision that's right for you. Do all of the above and then listen to your heart. Once you make a decision, make a commitment to make it work. Then take action to make it happen, even a small step in the right direction.

Risk Avoidance

Whether or not you consider yourself a risk taker, you take risks every day in the course of your life and work. There are risks associated with everything you do. You can't avoid risks; you can only minimize them. How? By getting as much information as you can, talking to experienced, knowledgeable people, doing some soul searching, and considering what you hope to gain from any situation. Why take risks at all? Because they create opportunities, vitality, and energy in your career, and are a necessary step to reaching your full potential.

When considering taking any career risks, whether changing specialties, quitting your job, taking a higher level position, or taking on more responsibility, ask yourself, "What's the worst that can happen if I do this?" Examples: "I could hate it; I could not do as well at it as I was hoping; I might not get along with the people; I might miss my current coworkers." Then also ask yourself "What's the best that could happen if I do this?" Examples: "I could love it; I could excel at it; It could lead to other things; I can grow and utilize more of my potential and talents; I could make some great contacts and some new friends." You've heard the expression, "Nothing ventured, nothing gained." Although the lure of the comfort zone is strong, there is no progress without some intelligent risk taking.

Other benefits can only be realized once you take the risks. Remember the job I took with the company that did medical exams for insurance companies? I took a significant risk in accepting that position on many levels. I left the relative security of a cushy job with a good company to do something totally different. I also took a significant pay cut to work there. I knew that the job offered avenues for learning and the type of low-key environment and work schedule I was looking for. I couldn't possibly have known that a brand new system of healthcare reimbursement (the DRG system) would be implemented while I was working there, and that I would have an opportunity to be trained in its use. Yet, that turned out to be one of the biggest opportunities of my career which led me to a position in a hospital where I first began to form my vision of becoming a public speaker and a career coach. Was I simply lucky? Luck had nothing to do with it. This is the type of thing that happens when you get yourself out there, move forward in your career, make decisions, and take calculated career risks.

Keep in mind that there is no failure, only different lessons to learn. Concentrate less on the outcome and more on the experience. Joy and benefits come from just doing and trying. Not everything is about outcomes. Focus on the journey. It is all part of the process of learning, growing, and moving forward.

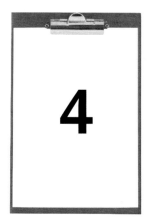

Looking for Your Next Job

W hether in the job market by choice or necessity, job-finding basics are the same. And while most people usually look for employment in print or online ads, there are many other, often more effective ways, to find and land a good job.

Networking — Your Best Choice

In chapters 2 and 3, we discussed networking to explore career options, to obtain information about specialties, and to stay connected. Networking is also one of the best and most effective ways to find and get a good job. Fifty to 90% of all jobs are found through networking or "word of mouth." Personal contacts and connections are your best source when in the job market. Does that mean you have to personally know someone in a particular specialty or who works for a company to get in? Not at all. Chances are that someone you know knows someone else, who knows someone else who can put you in touch with someone who does. The more people you talk to, the larger your network becomes.

You may have heard someone say, "I got this job through dumb luck. It just fell into my lap. I was talking to my neighbor when he mentioned his company was looking for a nurse." That's not dumb luck, that's networking. Sometimes you may initiate the networking contacts; other times, contacts may come to you. The process works rather well, which is why you should always stay connected and visible. It's who you know, and who knows you that will contribute to your success.

Networking for a job involves launching a targeted campaign to connect with those you already know, to make new strategic contacts, and to cultivate ongoing relationships, with old and new contacts. It also involves becoming visible through professional and social channels. Networking will help you uncover unadvertised jobs, provide introductions to decision makers, and provide insider information on an industry, positions, companies, salaries, and other employment information.

So, how can you use networking in the job search process? Let's count the ways.

First Things First

Networking with the objective of job-seeking uses strategies that go beyond networking to merely stay connected. A business card is one fundamental to any networking situation, but particularly vital when looking for a job. (See Chapter 10.) Even if you're currently employed and have a business card related to your present position, you should have a generic card with personal contact information just for networking. This way people can contact you outside of work and long after you've left your current employment. Remember to carry those cards with you wherever you go because you never know who you'll meet.

Who Ya Gonna Call?

The easiest way to launch your networking campaign is to get on the telephone and start contacting former coworkers and supervisors, nursing instructors and colleagues, physicians, and others who know you. Don't limit your contacts to healthcare workers since everyone has connections in different industries. The power of networking is that people know people who know other people, in all walks of life.

If you haven't spoken to any of your contacts in a while, take a minute to catch up. Ask them how they're doing and ask what they've been up to. Let them know you're alive and well and in the job market. If there's something specific you're interested in, say so. For example, "I'm looking to get into research working for a pharmaceutical company," or "I'm looking to transition into labor & delivery."

If you don't know exactly what you want to do, you can let people know that you're in the market for "something different." Of course the more specific you are, the better. If you're not sure what you're looking for, then at least narrow your search. For instance, you might tell people that you do or don't want to work in a hospital, are looking for something you can do from home, or prefer a job dominated by computer work. You can also say something general, such as "I'm looking to do something different from what I've done in the past. I'd ideally like to work from home using my computer. Please keep your ears open for me. I'm exploring my options." Because you want to continuously expand your network, always add, "Do you know anyone else I might be able to speak with?" If they give you a contact, add, "May I say that you referred me?" Getting referrals is important because a mutual connection with someone you're contacting is better than contacting someone "cold." Use that connection when calling and writing by indicating who referred you or suggested the contact.

If you know what you want to do and happen to know someone who works in that industry, start there. For example, if you want to break into the pharmaceutical industry, you should contact anyone you know who is associated in any way with that industry, regardless of his or her position. Let

The Power of Networking

A nurse who had just relocated to my area recently contacted me. She wanted to work in a dermatology office in her new location. She heard me talk about the value of networking in job-hunting and called me for advice. She knew people who worked in dermatology in her old location, but she didn't know anyone here or how to start her networking. I told her to begin with connections from her former locale by letting them know where she was and what she was looking for. Perplexed, she responded, "But I want to work in this state, not in the one I just left." I explained that people have connections all over the country. Professional people join national associations and attend conventions. They probably have associates who have relocated themselves. I emphasized that networking does not have to be done only with people who directly work for a company or facility for which you wish to work or even in the same state. The power of networking knows no geographic boundaries. Just because people live elsewhere doesn't mean they don't have contacts and connections in other areas.

Remember, you shouldn't limit networking efforts to those who work in a particular specialty or even to those in healthcare. You never know who has a brother, cousin, or neighbor who works in the industry or for a company in which you want to be employed. The power of networking is so far-reaching that you should cast your net widely.

them know of your interest and ask for their help in achieving your goal. You might say something like, "I'm very interested in exploring a career in pharmaceutical research. I was hoping you could refer me to someone in the research department at your company. I'd also appreciate any advice you can give me about breaking into the field. I value your opinion."

If you wanted to change specialties and get into labor & delivery, for instance, it would make sense to talk to anyone you know who works in that specialty, regardless of their employer or location. How can acquaintances who work at other hospitals in other cities possibly help you get a position in a local hospital? They may be connected through professional associations, employers, and even through friends and family.

One of my favorite networking stories comes from a nurse who seized an opportunity on the very day she was attending one of my seminars. We were in a large city, and the group was on lunch break. During that time, this nurse was walking outside and saw a large group of people walking out of another hotel, all carrying canvas bags emblazoned with the logo of a well-known pharmaceutical company. Having just heard my spiel about networking, she decided to approach one member of the group. She said, "I couldn't help noticing your tote bags. I'm a nurse and have always been

Networking at Its Best

I once received a phone call from a nurse who had attended my Career Alternatives for Nurses® seminar. She was very excited and wanted to tell me about a positive networking experience.

"The weekend after your seminar, I attended a block party in my neighborhood. I remembered what you said about 'getting the word out' and decided to let those I spoke with know I was in the job market. I was talking to a man I knew through church. I'd heard he was an accountant, but I didn't know much else about him. In the course of conversation, I mentioned that I wanted to get into pharmaceutical research. He said, 'Really? I work for XXX Pharmaceutical Company. I could probably refer you to someone in the research department there.' I was dumb-struck for a moment, but then said, 'You're kidding. I thought you were an accountant.' He said, 'I am an accountant, but I happen to work for XXX.'" A week later this nurse had a job interview with this company and a month later, a job offer. She was astonished at how a casual conversation at a social function with someone she didn't know well could lead to such as incredible opportunity. That's networking at its best!

interested in working in your industry. The woman she approached was also a nurse, who said, "I'll be happy to help you, do you have a business card?" (Get those cards made!) She did not, but asked for the person's card and said she would contact her later. Opportunities are everywhere, if you just look for them.

Once you've made connections, stay in touch with them and keep them posted on your progress. Send a follow-up note after a meeting or a phone call and include your business card, even if you previously gave one. Having business cards in your contacts' hands or on their desks is a good way to keep you fresh in their mind. It's also necessary if they want or need to contact you or refer someone to you. Any correspondence you have with contacts should always include your full contact information. Don't make anyone work to get in touch with you. An e-mail follow-up is okay for networking encounters, but people appreciate a personalized hand written note.

Keep a notebook or index cards of your contacts, when and where you met them, and any advice or referrals they gave you. Stay organized and remember the origins of your leads so you can update and thank the right person afterwards.

Get Yourself Out There and Be Visible

Your job-hunting campaign should include getting out on a regular basis to career fairs, professional association meetings, nursing conventions, and conferences. In addition to nursing and healthcare career fairs, go to industry-specific career fairs, such as those run for the pharmaceutical and information technology (computer-related) industries. Consider also attending general career fairs, where all types of positions are made available, as there are invariably numerous healthcare facilities and companies exhibiting there. These events are advertised in trade publications and in such main-

Time Well Spent

I recently heard from a nurse who told me she always thought attending career fairs was a waste of time. After reading one of my articles, she decided to get out to a nursing career fair in her area. Later she informed me that she had found her dream job, an entry-level position doing a specialized type of case management, working for a private review company. You never know what will happen when you get yourself out there.

stream media as newspapers, radio, and the Internet. Opportunities are everywhere.

You should also attend open houses, open interviews, and recruitment events offered by prospective employers, even if you're not sure what they have to offer or whether you even want to work for them. Attending such events is a great way to learn more and make great contacts. You just never know what opportunities might present themselves. Remember that face-to-face networking is best and most effective.

Eight Steps to Maximize Your Time at a Career Fair or Convention

Dress to Impress: Make a good impression even if you're not actively looking for a job. Stand out from the crowd as a polished professional. Dress as you would for an interview (wear a suit or your best outfit — see Chapter 8). You'll make some of your most important professional contacts at these events and you want to look sharp.

Determine Your Objective: Consider what you want to accomplish while there. Are you seeking a job offer or exploring career options? Do you want to gather information about graduate schools? Are you seeking a personal connection with an editor or publisher who may be there? Think about what is most important to you and how your time will be best spent.

Scan the Exhibitors' List: Most events provide a list of exhibitors along with their location in the exhibit hall. Scan the list for those you'd most like to connect with and visit those booths first. This will ensure that you have sufficient time to make your most important contacts. You can use your remaining time to browse the exhibitor floor or visit secondary targets.

Make Personal Contacts: Approach selected exhibitors with direct eye contact and a smile. Introduce yourself with a full, firm handshake. Ask about the company/facility they represent and inquire about what opportunities exist there for nurses, if appropriate. Remember, these events are not just for job hunting. You're gathering information and making important contacts.

Carry Business Cards: Personal or work-related business cards are a great way to exchange contact information and are essential for professional networking.

Informational Interviewing

An informational interview, also known as an information-gathering interview, is a more formalized type of networking. It involves a formal interview, that is, talking in a structured way to someone who works in a specialty you are interested in or for a company you wish to work for.

Informational interviewing is an effective way to learn more about a particular specialty and position. It's a good way to get inside information

• •

See Chapter 10 for the whys and how-tos of creating and carrying cards. Some nurses also carry preprinted address labels to save time when wishing to add their contact information to the mailing list of selected vendors.

Follow-Up: Always reinforce your initial contacts by sending a note or making a phone call. Let them know you enjoyed meeting them and follow up on anything discussed. Because this is not an interview follow-up, it would be appropriate to send an e-mail or hand-written follow-up note here.

Be sure to ask for the card of anyone you wish to stay in touch with or may want to contact at a later date. To jog your memory later, jot down on the back of their cards where and when you met them and any important issues discussed.

Bring Your Résumé: Regardless of your purpose in attending, it is always wise to bring updated copies of your résumé to these events. You never know what might come up or who will request a copy. Even if you're happily employed, you may discover an opportunity to do some consulting on the side, some writing or teaching, or even learn of a career opportunity that you never considered. It's best to be prepared.

Act Professional: While it's OK to avail yourself of some of the free samples offered by vendors, such as pens and candy, it is appropriate to first make eye contact with, and greet the vendor before taking anything. It's also polite to ask first, too, since everything on the table is not necessarily a free sample. Some vendors have had books and tapes that were for sale as well as their own personal pens and mugs taken by overzealous attendees. Likewise, it is appropriate to take one of something that is offered for free, not a handful, unless otherwise indicated.

• •

about a company or industry, too. It can yield advice about breaking into that industry or specialty as well as provide specific contacts. Informational interviewing is an effective method of gaining access to a decision maker in a company and other influential people in a particular specialty. It can also be a great way to get your foot in the door somewhere.

Informational interviewing is an indirect and effective way of finding a job. In the course of conducting the interview and making the contact, you may uncover unadvertised jobs in that company, obtain a referral for a job in another company, or even be offered a job. Since the major objective of an informational interview is to get information, advice, and additional contacts, you should not ask for a job. However, if one is offered, that would be a bonus. Informational interviewing is a valuable networking tool even if you are not yet actively seeking employment, but simply exploring options.

Here's how it works: Make a list of people you'd like to talk to, and not necessarily people you already know. You could list people who work in a particular industry, who are doing something you'd like to do, people you admire, or who you'd like to work for. The list might include officers of a related professional association at state, national, or local levels. For example, if you were considering getting into infection control, you might arrange an informational interview with the state chapter president of the Association for Professionals in Infection Control and Epidemiology.

While informational interviewing can be done by telephone, or e-mail if necessary, an in-person meeting is always preferable and should be your objective. That is because, as previously mentioned, face to face networking is more powerful than any other method. The opportunity to meet, shake hands, and interact with someone up close and personal is the most effective approach you can use. Of course, if the person you wish to speak with is not geographically near you, a telephone interview will suffice. When arranging for a telephone interview, ask the person if they prefer to get the questions ahead of time by e-mail.

Make initial contact with each person by telephone or with a letter of introduction (see example). E-mail can be used for an initial contact to set up an appointment to speak further. However, a hard copy letter in the mail, such as the one mentioned above, is preferable because it is more formal and allows you to carefully state your interest and intent. A formal letter would always be followed-up by a phone call.

If making an initial contact by phone, be prepared with what you want to say. Start with a brief introduction and then be sure the person is free to speak with you briefly. Say something like, "Hi, Ms. Arnold. My name is

Carol Jenkins, and I'm a registered nurse interested in learning more about psychiatric nursing. Do you have a moment to speak with me?" If Ms. Arnold says yes, then you can continue with something like, "I'd love the opportunity to meet with you in person to ask you some questions about psychiatric nursing and to learn more about you and how you got into your current position." If Ms. Arnold were to say, "Are you looking for a job because we don't have any openings right now," you might respond by saying, "That's not why I'm calling you. I'm looking for some information and advice."

Ms. Arnold might then respond by saying, "Well, can't we do this over the phone?" Since your objective is to get an in-person meeting, you might say something like, "We could, but I've prepared a résumé and would appreciate it if you could look it over and give me some advice." If Ms. Arnold says, "Well why don't you fax it to me?" you could counter with, "I could do that, but I know that the overall appearance of my résumé, as well as the content, is important. Besides, I would be thrilled to meet you face-to-face and have an opportunity to speak to you in-person." That approach is hard to resist. In other words, be persuasive and overcome objections to get that meeting. You may have to sell the idea to some people, but believe me, it will pay off for you.

In spite of your best efforts, there will always be some people who can't or won't agree to meet you in person for a variety of reasons. Perhaps they are overloaded with work, have personal challenges, or are trying to meet a deadline. In that case, try to at least get some phone time from them. Be prepared with your questions whenever you call someone in case they say, "Gee I'd love to meet with you, but we're being surveyed in a month, and I just can't spare the time. However I have a few moments now if you want to ask me some questions," or, "If you send me your questions by e-mail, I'll answer them when I have a few moments." Take whatever you can get. On the rare occasion that you encounter someone who seems put off by your request, thank them for their time, wish them a good day, and move on to your next contact.

Always set a specific time frame for the meeting and stick to it. For example, you might say or write, "I'll only take 20 minutes of your time." If they say, "I can only give you 15 minutes," take it. For an in-person interview, dress as you would for a job interview. (See Chapter 8.) Bring a small notebook with you and have your questions written down so you don't forget anything. It is perfectly appropriate to take notes during the interview, just don't write non-stop since you want to have eye contact and some personal interaction with the individual. You want them to get to know you, too.

Questions to ask —

- How did you get started in the specialty?
- What do you like most/least about your job?
- What is the job outlook for the next five years in this specialty/industry?
- Can you describe a typical day?
- Are there any industry trends I should know about?
- What professional associations do you or others in this specialty belong to?
- What are typical salary ranges in this specialty for entry-level and advanced positions?
- What advice do you have for someone interested in breaking into the specialty?
- How do you see someone like me fitting into this specialty?
- Do you know anyone else I can talk to? (If yes) Can I say that you referred me?

After the interview, whether it was by phone, e-mail, or in-person, send a thank you note. Thank the person for their time, sage advice, and insights. Then stay in periodic touch with them. If they gave you a lead or referral, follow-up with them and let them know how you made out. Keep them posted on your progress and do let them know when you find a position. A networking thank-you note can be hand-written or word-processed. However, since an informational interview is a more formal type of networking, I recommend sending a word-processed letter on good stationery but do use your judgment here. Whether hand-written or typed, the important thing is that you send the note.

Common Misgivings

You may be hesitant to approach people with this method because you are not accustomed to asking for help. Asking for help is not a sign of weakness, as many fear. Rather, it is a sign that you are intelligent, assertive, and humble enough to know you have a lot to learn.

You might also be asking yourself, "Why would a total stranger want to help me?" Contrary to what you might believe, most people have a natural instinct to want to help others. Most people are sincerely glad to be of assistance if approached in the right manner. When you approach someone with courtesy and respect, show interest in them and their specialty, and exhibit enthusiasm, you will be surprised at how total strangers will bend over backwards to help you. Why? For some people it is an ego boost to be sought out for advice. Others will identify with your situation and remember when they were first getting started. The latter is certainly true for me. I am always happy to give advice or guidance to someone who asks. Many others helped me along the way, and I am only too happy to pass that on. Most people feel that way. That's what makes the world go round.

Networking is unquestionably the best and most effective way to find a job. But a successful job search campaign will employ many different strategies for maximum benefit. Here are several more.

The Want Ads

The want ads, also known as the classified ads, are the most commonly used, yet the least effective method of finding jobs. Estimates are that only 5% to 10% of all available jobs ever get into the classifieds. That's probably surprising to those of you who rely so heavily on them. The higher the level and more desirable the position, the less likely it is to appear in the classifieds. Why? These positions are filled primarily through word of mouth and other means, which we'll discuss in a moment.

However, don't ignore the want ads because they can lead to some interesting positions. They can also open doors of opportunity and uncover unadvertised or "hidden" jobs as they did for me early in my career. There are multiple sources of classified ads so be sure to explore them all. Here are the most common ones:

Nursing and healthcare magazines: Targeted classifieds, such as those found in industry journals, can yield some good information. In addition to general nursing magazines, be sure to check the classified ads in nursing and healthcare publications specifically geared to managers and administrators. Also, use specialty journals for related classified ads. For example, if you were looking for a position in occupational health nursing, you'd want to check out the ads in the *AAOHN Journal,* the official publication of the American Association of Occupational Health Nurses. You can find these publications in the medical library of a local hospital, or you can find them in the periodical section of a college that offers degrees in nursing or healthcare.

Public newspapers: Be sure to check the large circulation newspapers in your area, including those of nearby big cites. For example, if you want to work in New Jersey, you would naturally check the New Jersey newspapers.

However, *The New York Times* and *The Philadelphia Inquirer* also carry ads for positions in New Jersey because of their proximity to the state.

Don't just look in the "Healthcare" section of the ads, either. Some companies will post relevant positions under headings, such as "Sales," "Medical," "Computers," and others. Be sure to look in the large display ads in the front of the classified section, too.

The Internet: The Internet is a rapidly expanding, vast source of classified ads. You'll find job postings on career-related websites, professional association websites, company/facility websites, and employment/nursing agency websites. Many newspapers and magazines also post their print want ads on their website. Even though the Internet seems like a convenient and abundant source of ads, keep in mind that these are still classified ads and as such, only represent a small percentage of all available jobs. We'll discuss posting your résumé online in Chapter 6.

Again, that may yield you some job prospects, but your time could be better spent by getting on the telephone and networking or getting out to some career events or conventions. Relying solely on your "paperwork" to sell you is one of the toughest ways to find and get a job.

Attitude Is Everything

Read want ads with a grain of salt. Often the specifications in an ad are not set in stone and are more flexible than the average reader realizes. Ads that state certain credentials or experience are 'desirable,' 'preferred,' 'ideal' or 'a plus' only means it would be nice but isn't necessary. Even if an ad says that something is 'required,' that point is often more negotiable than you might think. If you see an ad that appeals to you, you should give it your best shot.

Several years ago, I met a young nurse who had recently graduated from an associate degree program. She was interested in research and applied for a part-time research position she saw advertised at a local university. The ad stated that all candidates must have at least three years of clinical experience and a minimum of a bachelor's degree, master's degree preferred. This recent graduate nurse did not meet any of those specifications but applied for the job anyway. She was offered the job and happily accepted. How could this happen? Because when all is said and done, prospective employers are looking to hire a personality, not just a body to fill a slot. This young nurse was personable, professional, and enthusiastic about research. Attitude is everything.

Keep in mind that want ads are known as "open jobs." That means they are publicly advertised, so often there are many applicants representing a lot of competition for the same job. We'll discuss cover letters in Chapter 6. Many more effective and direct approaches can be used to uncover unadvertised jobs, such as making direct contact with prospective employers. Here are a few ways to do that.

Direct Mail Campaign

A direct mail campaign involves sending a letter of introduction and interest to a specific company or person you'd like to work for (see example). It is a targeted job search technique used to uncover unadvertised jobs in a particular company or industry and to gain access to industry leaders. The approach is somewhat different from requesting an informational interview in that you are directly asking for a job. For example, if you wished to work for a healthcare information technology company or wanted to break into quality improvement, you would target certain companies and facilities that might offer these positions. You would then identify a decision maker for the specific department or division you'd like to work for; that is, someone who has the authority to actually hire you. This might be a department director, a division manager, a vice president, a regional director, etc.

Let's say you wanted to get into quality improvement. You would target healthcare facilities, insurance companies, and private review companies that offer such positions. You would then identify a decision maker in a related department, such as the Director of Quality Improvement. You can identify the decision makers in a particular company by asking around, looking at company websites, or calling the company or department directly. You might contact a local hospital and say, "Could you please give me the name and title of the person in charge of the quality improvement department?" Hopefully, the person answering the phone will have that information or will transfer you to someone who does. Be sure to get the exact spelling of the person's name, his or her exact title, and any credentials if applicable (e.g., RN, PhD, etc.). If you are asked why you want the information, you can simply say, "I want to send them something in the mail," which is true. Do not say you are looking for a job because you will be put through to human resources instead.

If you've decided you wanted to work for a particular product company, such as one that makes computer software for nurses or one that makes monitors or respirators, decide what capacity you want to work in and then identify the appropriate decision maker. For example, are you interested in sales or marketing vs. training and development, or do you wish to work as a clinical consultant? If you're not sure, do some informational interviewing first.

Marketing Letter Basics

Marketing letters should be sent to those who have direct authority to hire you, not to human resources. That is because any human resource department receives dozens and sometimes hundreds of résumés each day for a wide variety of positions. It may take time for the clerical staff to sort and screen those résumés and see that they get to the right person. Not only do you have additional people scrutinizing your résumé, but this way, the more people who handle it, the more likely it is to get lost or misrouted. With the direct mail approach, you are bypassing the human resource department and going directly to the decision maker.

There are two schools of thought on whether or not to include your résumé with a marketing letter. On the one hand, if a résumé falls out of the envelope, the correspondence may look too much like a job application and the receiver may automatically pass it on to human resources for processing without reading the letter. Therefore, if there is no résumé enclosed, you may increase the likelihood of your letter being read and considered. It can serve to whet the reader's appetite and leave him or her wanting more information. Of course, you would have highlighted your relevant experience in your letter. On the other hand, if a prospective employer is intrigued by your letter, he or she may be frustrated or annoyed that you have not included your résumé with additional details about your background. Consider both perspectives when deciding whether to send a résumé or not on the initial contact.

Every marketing letter must be followed-up with a phone call. Don't even bother to send them out if you don't intend to do this. Remember, you're asking the prospective employer for a job so you need to remain proactive in the situation. Don't just throw the ball into their lap and expect them to act on it. You want something from them and have to pursue it. End every marketing letter with a statement indicating that you will call in a week as follow-up (refer to example).

When you make the follow-up call, several things may happen. You might get a 'gatekeeper,' such as a receptionist or staff member. In a very assertive voice say something like, "Hi. Carol Roberts calling for Janet Fredericks. Is she in?" If you are asked, "Is she expecting your call?" You would say, "Yes," because you had stated you would call in your letter. If asked what this is in reference to, you can state that it is a follow-up to some correspondence you had sent her last week.

If Ms. Fredericks is not in or available, rather than automatically leaving a message, ask, "When is a good time to reach her?" Don't leave a message right away expecting her to call you back. Remember what I said about staying proactive in the situation? Determine another time to call and try again. Likewise, if you keep getting voice mail or an answering machine, don't leave a message right away. Keep calling back on different days and times in an effort to reach her. Try calling before 9 AM and after 5 PM. Many managers and directors are in early and stay late. If the regular office staff is not there, managers and directors will often answer their own telephone.

If you call repeatedly and can't get through to the person you want to speak to, leave a message and state a specific day and time you will call back. For example, you might say, "This is Janet Roberts calling. I sent you a letter last week about my interest in working for you. I've been trying to reach you all week without success. I know you are very busy, so I will try you again this Thursday at 4 PM. If you care to speak with me in the interim, I can be reached at (phone #)." Speak slowly, clearly, and distinctly. Sound assertive and upbeat. Leaving a message indicating a specific day and time for a callback demonstrates a seriousness of purpose on your part and the recipient is more inclined to take your call or leave a message for you. Of course you do have to call back when you said you would, or you blow your credibility.

Once you reach Ms. Fredericks, introduce yourself briefly and refresh her memory as to who you are. You might say, "Hi, Ms. Fredericks. My name is Janet Roberts. I'm the critical care nurse who wrote to you last week, telling you how much I'd like to work for you. Do you have a moment to speak with me?" If she says, 'Yes,' be ready with a short statement requesting a meeting with her to further discuss your mutual interests. Then stop talking and let her respond. If she says there are no openings now but she'll keep you in mind, say, "I appreciate that. In the meantime, I'd love to meet you and learn more about you and how you got started in this field. I'd also be grateful if you could look over my résumé and give me a few tips on breaking into this field." In other words, you should not let a great opportunity to connect with this person slip through your fingers just because there are no jobs available. Even if no job is available, he or she may be able to help you in other ways. Go back to the steps for setting up and conducting an informational interview and take it from there.

Marketing letters can be particularly useful when trying to break into a new specialty or industry and as an adjunct to other job finding methods. Do keep in mind that one on one networking is still your best approach in all situations. Now let's look at some methods for getting a third party involved in your job search.

Getting Some Help

There are a number of different types of firms and agencies that match job seekers with employers. Although the term "recruiter" is used in many different settings, there is a difference between the types of agencies they work for and the types of positions and companies they work with. Here are several different categories of organizations and individuals you might seek out to assist you in the job search process.

Professional Recruiters

These individuals, commonly referred to as professional recruiters, headhunters, and search consultants, search for qualified people to fill specific job openings for client companies. The firm they own or work for is known as a search firm. You might use this type of firm to find a management, administrative, or education position. You might also use this type of firm to find a nontraditional position, such as one in nursing informatics, healthcare sales and marketing, quality improvement, medical writing, case management, etc. You would generally not use this type of firm to find a direct patient care position at the staff nurse level.

Here's how professional recruiters work. Their client is a company or agency/facility that has a professional position that needs to be filled. The recruiter contracts with that company to find qualified individuals based on the client's specifications. The recruiter will then scout around for candidates, screen them, and assemble one or more individuals to send on an interview with the client.

Professional recruiters locate candidates primarily by putting the word out to their network. However, you may receive a phone call from recruiters who are looking for a particular type of candidate. I have heard nurses say, "How did they get my name?" or, "How did they find me?" Professional recruiters will sometimes call all area hospitals or healthcare facilities to speak with nurses in similar positions to those they are working on. If you post your résumé online, you may also receive communication from professional recruiters. They may occasionally place a "blind" ad for the position in a newspaper looking for qualified candidates. A 'blind' ad is one in which no company name appears. A recruiter's ad might read something like, "RN with management experience needed for facility director's position with large metropolitan hospital. Salary range 80K to 90K (indicating that the salary is in the $80,000 to $90,000 range)." At the bottom of the ad it may say, "Qualified candidates contact the Henderson Agency," although in some cases, there may only be a PO Box or fax number.

A recruiter will screen potential candidates by phone and possibly in person if the recruiter and candidate are geographically near one another. Once the candidate is deemed qualified, the recruiter will set up an interview for the candidate with the client. The recruiter becomes a go-between for the prospective employer and the job candidate. This means that the job candidate communicates primarily with the recruiter before and after interviews unless otherwise specified.

There are a number of advantages to working with professional recruiters. These recruiters often have access to hidden jobs, those that are not publicly advertised. A recruiter has in-depth knowledge of what his or her client is looking for and will likely share that information with you. This information can be very helpful during the interview process. A recruiter will usually coach you in the interview process and may even role-play with you to help you deal with challenging questions or potential objections. He or she may even critique your résumé. Additionally, a recruiter will often negotiate salary and benefits for you with the client so you do not have to be directly involved with the company. Just like real estate agents, recruiters are skilled negotiators and can help to seal the deal.

Early in my career, I met a woman who was a recruiter of sales and marketing professionals. She was working on several related positions in the healthcare industry, and she encouraged me to come and talk to her further. I wasn't sure that healthcare sales and marketing was the right direction for me but decided to see how things went. The recruiter sent me on an interview for a company that manufactures respirators. She critiqued my résumé, coached me on what to wear, how to act, and even gave me tips on probable questions I would be asked and how to answer them. This was a great help since I had never been on a "corporate" interview before. The interview went well, and I was asked back for a second interview, but I decided not to pursue it further. However, it was a great learning experience for me, and I sharpened my interview skills in the process.

After you've been on an interview, the prospective employer will give the recruiter some feedback. The recruiter will likely share that information with you. This can be very helpful in the event of a subsequent interview or in the process of perfecting your self-presentation skills. You'll have a good idea of where you stand and what you need to do to move forward. Remember, the recruiter is motivated to help you get the job. Recruiters don't make any money unless they successfully "place" someone in a position (More on that in a moment). Another advantage to working with recruiters is that you can get some great interview experience whether you take a job through them or not.

You may be wondering why a company would choose to work with a recruiter rather than fill the position themselves. There are several possible reasons. A company may want to conduct a discreet job search. That is, they may not want the position to be publicly advertised for a variety of reasons. They may not want their competitors to know of the opening, or they may not want their own staff to know of the opening. In some cases, a company simply doesn't want to go through the hassle of advertising for a position, screening candidates, etc. They leave that up to the professional recruiter who will just be sending them pre-screened candidates for interviews.

Some additional things to know about working with professional recruiters —

Most professional recruiters specialize. They either work within a particular industry and/or with a particular type of position. For example, some recruiters work exclusively with sales and marketing positions, including healthcare sales and marketing. Other recruiters work primarily with nursing management positions or healthcare management in general, both in and out of the hospital. Some recruiters work exclusively with the pharmaceutical industry, information technology industry, or managed care industry.

You are not obligated to take any job you interview for when you work with a recruiter. Of course you should be earnest in your interest and pursuit, but if a job is not right for you, you can say so. It would not be ethical to then directly approach that company about employment for that same position in an effort to circumvent the recruiter. Nor would it be ethical to refer a friend to that company. For that reason, a recruiter may not reveal the name of a client until he or she is ready to send you on an interview. Recruiters are not being cagey or secretive. They are simply protecting their own interests.

The recruiter makes money by receiving a fee from the client — the employer — once the recruiter has successfully placed a candidate in

that position. A recruiter's fee is usually a percentage of the salary the candidate is hired at, although sometimes other arrangements are made. For example, if you were hired at $80,000, and the recruiter had an agreement with the client to place a candidate for 20% of the annual starting salary, the recruiter would receive a fee of $16,000 for the service. Some recruiters are paid a retainer fee, rather than a commission, for the service they provide.

You should never pay a fee to a professional recruiter. In fact, this is actually illegal in many cases. You should also be wary of a recruiter that offers additional services for a fee, such as résumé writing, interview coaching, or career counseling. Many recruiters offer these services at no cost to job candidates.

Commonly Asked Questions

How Can I Locate a Professional Recruiter?

As with any profession, some recruiters are more reputable than others. Therefore, as with any professional services, the best way to locate an appropriate recruiter for your job search is through a personal referral or recommendation. That means you should ask people who work in the same profession and specialty area that you are looking to work within. Let's say you wanted to work within the information technology industry (a.k.a. computer industry) as a nursing informatics specialist. Ask anyone who works in the IT world who the good recruiters are in the industry. They'll likely know or be able to find out. Likewise, if you wanted to work in the pharmaceutical industry, you could ask any pharmacist or drug salesperson. Chances are these people know because recruiters are in touch with them periodically.

Professional recruiters generally do not advertise in the yellow pages. That is because they do not necessarily want people who are looking for a job calling them. That does not mean you cannot make direct contact with a recruiter you wish to work with, but we'll discuss that more in a moment. Occasionally, a recruiter will place an ad for his services in the back of select professional journals and publications, usually those geared more toward managers and administrators.

You can also find a book in the library or bookstores titled *The Directory of Executive Recruiters.* This resource book cross-references recruiters by geographic location and specialty or industry. Of course not every recruiter is listed in this book. You can also look on the Internet using search terms, such as "healthcare search firms" or "executive search firms," to locate some.

Some associations, such as The American Organization of Nurse Executives (www.aone.org), list some executive search firms on their websites.

Can I Work With More Than One Recruiter?

Yes, but not on the same job. It is possible that more than one search firm is working on the same professional opportunity. For example, you may already be interviewing, or being considered, for a position with a particular company through a search firm. You might be contacted by another search firm who discusses a certain position they are conducting a search for without mentioning the company/facility name. The position sounds very similar to one you are already interviewing for. You should say something to the recruiter like, "Is this by any chance a position with County Medical?" The recruiter will either confirm that it is that position or advise you that it is not. If it is the same, you should advise this recruiter that you are already being considered for that position through another search firm.

A recruiter may ask you to enter into an exclusive arrangement with them — meaning you would not work with other search firms during a specified period of time. While you are under no obligation to do so, it can work to your advantage to agree to a short-term exclusivity contract of not more than two weeks. When you agree to this, the recruiter will often work extra hard during that time to find an appropriate position for you.

How Do I Approach a Recruiter I'd Like to Work With?

Once you've received a referral to, or recommendation for a particular recruiter or you've identified who you want to contact, make an initial phone call or send an e-mail. Introduce yourself, and explain what you're interested in. For example, you might say something like, "My name is Frank Miller. I'm a registered nurse interested in getting into healthcare sales and marketing. I think we might be able to help each other. Do you have a few moments to speak with me?" Be clear, concise, and direct in your communication. Be ready to sell yourself and tell the recruiter what distinguishes you from the crowd.

This would be the wrong way to approach a professional recruiter: "Hi, I'm an RN and I'm looking to do something different outside of the hospital." The recruiter would likely say, "Well, what are you looking to do?" And you answer, "I'm really not sure. I kinda want to see what's out there." That's a sure way to turn the recruiter off. In other words, you have to have some concept of what you're looking for or at least sound like you do.

If you're speaking to a recruiter who specializes in healthcare management positions and you're not sure what you're looking for, say something like, "I'm particularly interested in education positions but will consider any management level position." You must master assertive telephone skills. And since professional recruiters all have their own specialties, it is also helpful to add, after stating your interests and background, "Are you the right recruiter to speak with?" If they say they are not, ask them for a referral to another, better suited, recruiter.

If working with a professional recruiter does not sound like the right choice for your job search, you still have other options for getting some help, including using staffing and employment agencies.

Staffing/Employment Agencies

There are many types of agencies, different from search firms that you might work with in seeking employment. Through these agencies, nurses can find per diem, part-time, temporary, contract, and even direct hire employment. Individuals who work in this industry may refer to themselves as recruiters, employment counselors, placement counselors, employment consultants, and staffing coordinators. Here are examples of different types of agencies.

Traditional nursing/healthcare staffing agencies. These agencies typically focus on nursing staffing in healthcare facilities and offer per diem and contract work. However, many staffing agencies also offer positions in alternate settings, such as school nursing, occupational health nursing, legal nurse consulting, nursing informatics, and others. Be sure to specifically ask about those other opportunities if you're interested in them.

Travel nurse agencies. Travel nurse agencies contract with nurses to take temporary assignments, on average three months in length at a time, in various parts of the country. Nurses can generally pick their own assignment regarding specialty and geographic location. Most travel nurse agencies will assist you in moving, finding housing, and getting a license to practice in your new location. I once met a nurse who worked for a travel nurse agency but only took assignments in her local area so she didn't have to travel at all. Of course, most nurses who work for travel nurse agencies do so because of the travel opportunity. Some agencies offer domestic as well as international assignments. For overseas assignments, the time commitment is longer, usually six months to two years in length.

Part-time and temp healthcare agencies. Some healthcare employment agencies specialize exclusively in part-time and temporary or "temp" work. Generally speaking, their focus is on positions away from the bedside, such as school nursing, occupational and public health nursing, opportunities in the pharmaceutical industry, etc. A temp job could last for a few days to a year.

For those nurses specifically looking for part-time and occasional work in a nontraditional setting, this type of agency can be helpful. The advantage of working with a part-time/temp agency in particular is that it is a good opportunity to try out a nontraditional specialty to determine if you like it before making a full-time commitment. Also, it's a great way to gain some experience and get your foot in the door of a company or industry you'd like to transition into. Even if you are looking for full-time employment, many part-time and temp jobs turn into full-time or lead to other full-time positions within the company. So if, for example, you are considering working in occupational health or pharmaceutical research, but either can't get your foot in the door anywhere, or would like to try it before applying for a full-time job, part–time, or temp employment through an agency is a good option.

General employment agencies. In addition to nursing and healthcare staffing agencies, there are some general employment agencies that occa-

Helen is a recruiter with 20 years experience in the employment industry, who works with both healthcare and non-healthcare job candidates. She offers the following advice to nurses:

- Appreciate the value you bring to the bigger healthcare industry. Some nurses come to me with no confidence in themselves. They undervalue their own skills and abilities and how those skills can be used in other industries and other settings beyond the hospital.

- If you get blown off by a company you wish to work for, ask if they use temps or consultants. If they say they do, ask, "Which agency do you work with?" Temping is a great way to get a foot in the door and gain valuable experience.

- When working with an agency, be flexible with your expectations and be open-minded about opportunities and salaries. Some candidates are very rigid and say, "This is who I am, and this is what I want." You may be cutting yourself off from some great opportunities.

sionally have positions for healthcare professionals, both permanent and temporary. Be sure to explore all sources.

The best way to find an agency of any type is through referral or word of mouth. Ask around and see who has worked with which agencies. Of course, most nursing agencies advertise in nursing publications and online. You can also look in the yellow pages of your phone book under "Nurses" and "Employment Agencies." And don't forget that agencies of all types exhibit at career and job fairs and conventions. It's a great chance to get up close and personal with recruiters.

Almost all nurse staffing agencies, including travel nurse agencies, require that a nurse have at least one year to two years of general patient care experience. That is because an agency nurse needs to hit the ground running in any assignment, adapt quickly to a new environment, and be able to work very independently. There is no orientation or preceptor and sometimes limited access to support systems. While new graduate nurses might be able to find nontraditional nursing work through an agency, they would not be qualified for a traditional patient care assignment here.

Many healthcare facilities and companies have their own in-house recruiters who recruit for all levels of positions within the company while others recruit for specific types of positions only. This includes hospitals, pharmaceutical companies, and others. If there are particular facilities/companies you wish to work for, try making direct contact with that recruiter via telephone or e-mail.

While recruiters work on connecting prospective employees with employers, some firms can facilitate the job search process in other ways.

Career Management/Outplacement Firms

We discussed career management services in Chapter 3 in relation to helping you decide what you want to do. Outplacement firms, career coaches, and counselors do not place you in positions but can assist you in the job search process. They may even have important contacts to help you along. Just be sure to understand the difference between a professional recruiter and agency who will directly hook you up with employers at no cost to you, as opposed to a career management firm that will primarily assist you with self-marketing and career focus for a fee, unless that fee is paid by your employer as the result of a lay-off or facility closing.

Using Volunteering as a Job Search Tool

By now you've noticed that various career management tools and techniques have more than one purpose. The same holds true for volunteering. Not only can volunteering provide some great experience, it can also be an effective job finding tool. If there is a specialty or an employer you really want to work for but haven't had any luck with through traditional channels, consider offering to volunteer there. Volunteering not only provides an opportunity to gain relevant experience, but it often leads to paid employment. Here are some real life examples of how other nurses used volunteering, some unwittingly, to land the job of their dreams.

Karen was a staff nurse for 15 years. She had done some career research and decided that she wanted to break into quality improvement. She applied for a few job openings she saw advertised in the classified ads but wasn't getting any calls. She decided to approach the director of the Quality Improvement (QI) department in her current place of employment. She inquired about openings but was told none existed at present. So she offered to volunteer two hours per week for them. She agreed to do whatever was necessary, even filing and answering the phone. She was desperate to get any exposure she could to the specialty. Lo and behold, four months down the road, a full time position became available for a QI nurse. The job wasn't even advertised yet and was offered to Karen. Why? Because she was already there, they knew her, and the transition was a breeze. Karen happily accepted the position. Although she never expected a job offer when initially offering to volunteer, her initiative paid off in big dividends.

Alyce (not her real name) was a very accomplished nurse working in a very narrow and highly specialized field. While she gave me permission to tell her story, she asked that I not reveal her industry. She had worked in her specialty for many years, held leadership positions in her national professional association, and was once editor of her specialty journal. She had worked her way to the top of her field and was quite content. One day she was notified that her department was being eliminated and she was being laid off. "I never saw it coming," she said. "It felt like the rug had been pulled out from under me. I panicked, wondering where I could possibly go from here. There were so few good positions available in my specialty, and the thought of starting over again at my age (58 years) was unfathomable." Alyce had been unemployed for almost a year when she attended one of my Career Alternatives for Nurses® seminars.

Three months after the seminar, Alyce contacted me with some exciting news. "I would have never thought of using volunteering as a job search technique before coming to your seminar. And honestly, I didn't really believe it would work. But I took your advice and thought about my ideal work situation. There was a facility I had always dreamed of working for, so I decided to contact them about a position in my specialty. They didn't have any openings when I called, so I told them I'd like to volunteer there anyway. Here I was sitting at home doing nothing and not getting paid. I figured I might as well do something constructive and not get paid. They were rather startled by my offer and said no one had ever offered to volunteer there before." Alyce became a volunteer for four hours a week at her "dream employer." Three months later, a part-time position opened up, and it was automatically offered to Alyce. She was told that the job would likely turn into a full-time position by the end of the year. Needless to say, she was ecstatic.

Carrie was a registered nurse and certified personal trainer. When she contacted me, she had been working exclusively as a personal trainer for several years and wanted to also utilize her nursing background. I suggested she look into cardiac rehabilitation, which combines nursing and fitness. She was very interested in the prospect but didn't feel she could just jump back into the clinical arena after an absence of several years. So I suggested she volunteer at a cardiac rehab center for awhile to get her bearings as this is a low-risk way to re-enter healthcare. After a few months there, she was feeling comfortable and confident and applied for a position in the department. They were thrilled to have her, and she found a way to combine her two loves: fitness and nursing.

Some Additional Job Finding Tips

When actively seeking employment, it is necessary for prospective employers to be able to contact you easily. Therefore, it is highly advisable to have an e-mail account and answering machine on your phone or voice mail messaging. While these two things are standard for many, there are still some people who do not have one or both.

E-mail is such a popular form of communication and is often the easiest way to get in touch with a job applicant. If you don't have an e-mail address, you might give the impression that you're behind the times and out of step. Be sure to have an e-mail address that is neutral and professional such as Fmccarthy@nnn.net. Examples of unprofessional e-mail addresses are: hotchicknurse@nnn.net or poohbearkisses@nnn.net. Check your e-mail and phone messages often and be sure that either doesn't get full or start to reject incoming messages. If you have a spam filter on your e-mail account, be sure to scan rejected e-mails to be certain a legitimate message didn't get inadvertently bumped into that folder. It happens all the time.

If no one is home to accept a phone call, and you do not have an answering machine or voice mail to take a message, it can make prospective employers crazy if they're trying to reach you to set up an interview. If they call you even once, get no answer and have no capacity to leave a message, they may not call again.

Be sure to have a professional message on your answering machine, too, at least while you're in the job market. Playing music or reciting a poem, having your children speak the message in unison, or saying something glib can be a turnoff to someone who doesn't know you yet.

Sample Letter of Introduction for Informational Interviewing

Carl Frazier, RN
200 Main Street
Crystal Cave, NJ 88094
(732) 555-0986
cfrazier@nnn.net

May 7, 20__

Janet Fredericks, RN
Chief Nurse
State of New Jersey
Department of Health Affairs
Trenton, NJ 88007

Dear Ms. Fredericks,

Carol Edwards of County General Hospital suggested I contact you. She said you were tops in your field and would be a great person for me to speak with. Congratulations on your career success! Like you, I am a registered nurse with a pediatric background. I am exploring my career options and am interested in working for state government.

I would appreciate the opportunity to meet briefly with you in-person, at your convenience, and learn more about you and how you got started in your current career path. I'm also interested in learning more about what other nurses are doing in the Department of Health Affairs.

I will contact you in the next week in the hopes that we can set up an appointment. In the meantime, if you care to reach me, my cell phone is (732) 555-8994.

Sincerely,

Carl Frazier, RN

Carl Frazier, RN

Sample Marketing Letter

Carl Frazier, RN
200 Main Street
Crystal Cave, NJ 88094
(732) 555-0986
cfrazier@nnn.net

November 8, 20__

Frederick Castle
Director, Health Services
College Health Plan
44 Alleghany Road
West Crawford, TX 88094

Dear Mr. Castle,

I'm seeking an administrative level position with College Health Plan. As a healthcare professional, I appreciate the role that managed care plays in keeping their members healthy and well. Always looking to stay ahead of the curve, I realize that a large managed care company offers exactly the type of opportunities I am looking for. College Health Plan is a leader in the managed care industry, and I've got my sights set on being a part of that winning team.

I am a registered nurse with more than 20 years of progressive clinical and managerial experience. I have been involved in project management, human resource management, new program development, and services marketing. In addition to solid and diverse experience, I possess great problem-solving and conflict management skills. I also have an innate ability to motivate and energize those around me, and I am passionate about healthcare in general. I would be an asset to your company.

Not only would I relish the opportunity to work under an established industry leader like yourself, but I would be privileged to become a part of your dynamic and growing company. I will contact you within the next week so that we can discuss our mutual interests further.

Very Truly Yours,

Carl Frazier, RN

Carl Frazier, RN

Sample Marketing Letter

Janice Smith, RN
45 Lane Avenue
Smithville, NJ 00090
(732) 555-0220

October 30, 20__

Mary Harris, RN
Director of Quality Management
Allenwood Hospital
311 City Street
Allenwood, NJ 22536

Dear Ms. Harris,

I am interested in working for Allenwood Hospital as a Quality Improvement Coordinator. I am attracted by Allenwood Hospital's reputation for quality and service, and I am confident I can contribute to that.

As an RN with more than 15 years of critical care experience, I possess excellent clinical and managerial skills. I have also developed good communication skills while interacting with physicians, patients, and other healthcare professionals in a variety of situations. As a result of my committee work and my involvement in nursing quality improvement, I have developed a keen interest in hospital-wide quality management activities and have decided to pursue this career path.

In summary, I can offer you solid clinical experience, the ability to work well with all types of people, as well as energy and enthusiasm. I am willing to start in an entry-level position and learn from the bottom up. I am a quick study and determined to become an outcomes management professional.

I look forward to meeting with you so that we can discuss our mutual interests further. I will call you in one week to follow-up.

Sincerely,

Janice Smith, RN

Janice Smith, RN

Your Résumé

A résumé is a key self-marketing tool. Yet very few nurses have an effective one. Why? Many of us have never taken the time to learn the correct way to develop one. Also, many of us are intimidated by the process and are uncomfortable writing about ourselves in a positive way. Many nurses, especially those who have been in the same job for an extended period of time, have never had any type of résumé. There was a time when nurses didn't even need one. Our license to practice was all that was required to be hired. But, of course, those days are long gone and every nurse needs a professional résumé ready to go at a moments notice. Note: A résumé and curriculum vitae (CV) are two entirely different documents used in different settings. I'll discuss CVs in Chapter 6.

The purpose of a résumé is to highlight your more interesting, significant, and marketable skills and experiences. It is a synopsis of your credentials, achievements, skill set, and work history. It is a snapshot of your entire career. Therefore, the goal of effective résumé writing is to maximize your experience on paper and put your best foot forward. You do not need to enumerate everything you ever did or reveal everything there is to know about you. Rather, you want to develop a document that conveys the best of your background and presents it in the best possible light. You want to pique the reader's interest. Think of it as an advertisement for a product or service, where the selling points are highlighted, not all of the specifics.

Résumés are not used just for job changing. They may be requested when applying for a promotion or transfer, putting in a proposal to speak at a conference, applying for a position on the board of a professional association, submitting an article for publication, or various other reasons. And, as previously discussed, you may be very happily employed now, but you never know when your employment situation will change, your needs will change, or an opportunity will present itself that you had not previously considered. For example, you might have an opportunity to do some part-time consulting while you maintain your current position, and a prospective client or employer might want to see your résumé or keep a copy on file. The point is if someone asks you for your résumé, you want to have one ready, not be scrambling to develop one at the last minute only to find that your computer printer is out of ink. Besides, it makes sense to keep an up-to-date, written record of your work experience and accomplishments. It is so easy to forget what you've done otherwise, especially as the years pass. Imagine suddenly needing a résumé when you don't have a current one and having to recall and construct, on short notice, 10 years worth of accomplishments and experiences. It has happened to many of us, and it is not a pretty sight! Nor is the resulting résumé.

By now it should be clear that if you don't have a résumé, it is time to develop one. If you do have one, chances are it needs to be updated and reformatted to reflect current résumé writing standards and to best showcase your unique background. And while most people break into a cold sweat at the thought of having to develop a résumé, the process is actually much less difficult once you understand the purpose and learn the correct format and style of résumé writing. Let's review the basics.

Format

There are essentially three different types of résumés: chronological, functional, and combination. All three have a unique purpose and differ in the way that information is presented. Let's take a closer look at each.

Chronological

The chronological résumé (example #1) is the most commonly used and the one most people are familiar with. It focuses on work experience and starts with the current or most recent position and works its way back from there. It lists each job with several bullet points of related information. This is the type that is preferred by most recruiters and prospective employers. It tells a story and shows progression of employment history.

Functional

A functional résumé (example #2) shifts the focus to experience and downplays individual jobs and work history. For example, a functional résumé would group experience by categories such as: teaching, writing, researching, sales/marketing, and clinical, etc. It might also include a general category, "Selected Accomplishments," for those things that the writer wishes to highlight beyond the experience categories. This type of résumé is best used for someone with extensive, exceptional, or unique experience who has been out of the work force for a while or someone who is looking to totally change gears in their career, such as going from clinical work to education. A consultant who is working independently might also use it. A prospective client is more interested in a consultant's relevant work experience than in his or her work history.

A functional résumé might also be an option for someone with a very erratic work history who may need or want to shift the focus away from an employment record to his or her strengths and abilities. I do not mean to imply that the functional format should automatically be used in the above-mentioned examples or that everyone who has been out of the workforce for a while should use it. That simply is not the case. The point is that the functional format may be a useful alternative to the chronological format in certain situations.

The theory behind the functional format is that it forces the reader (recruiter, client, or prospective employer) to focus on experience rather than dates and length of employment. If you can impress the reader on page one with your experiences and accomplishments, by the time she gets to the second page, your work history becomes less important or, at the very least, is deemphasized. Of course this theory is debatable.

On the downside, because some people use the functional résumé to downplay a problematic work history, the functional format makes some prospective employers suspicious. And because many employers are simply accustomed to the chronological format and prefer it, they get annoyed with this format. The bottom line is, consider your own unique

I once coached a nurse who had been out of the workforce for 15 years while raising a family. Before that, she had exceptional work experience in management and education. She also had outstanding credentials and many impressive accomplishments. She was an ideal candidate for a functional résumé. We worked together to compose a dynamite document that highlighted her strengths while downplaying her absence from the workforce. This type of résumé not only made the nurse feel more confident, but it was effective in getting her several interviews and ultimately an excellent position as the director of educational services for a social service agency.

background and career goals, and choose the format that best serves your needs.

Combination

This is a combination of formats (example #3) that might be used by a consultant, for someone in a very specialized field, or with unique and extensive experience. It generally combines elements of the chronological and functional résumés as well as the CV and would be typically longer than the average résumé, which is one to two pages. A combination résumé could feasibly be three to four pages in length.

When I went into business as a speaker, writer, and consultant, I shifted to a combination style of résumé, a cross between a functional résumé and a CV. Neither format was exactly right for me, so I took elements of both to create a document that worked for me. My clients are interested in specific types of experiences I have (speaking, writing, teaching) rather than my employment history. However, a simple functional résumé would not do in my case because I also have numerous publications, speaking credentials, awards, and professional association involvement. I use a three-page combination format to best showcase my background and credentials.

Layout and Writing Style

Today's prospective employers visually scan, rather than read, résumés. This means they give it an initial quick look-over to see if some basic elements are there, or if anything of interest catches their attention. It is said that the average résumé reader scans a résumé in three seconds to 20 seconds. What can they glean in that short amount of time? If written and organized well, they should be able to tell if you have the basic experience and credentials they are looking for. At the very least, they should be intrigued enough to want to read or "scan" more.

With that in mind, you should create a résumé in a high-impact style, that is, one that is well organized, concise, upbeat, and laid out to make information easy to find and 'scan' and hopefully read. The layout of your résumé should be consistent throughout the document.

The following are important characteristics of a high impact style of writing:

Use a Bulleted Format: Each piece of information or sound bite in the "Experience" section (or "Selected Accomplishments" section of a functional résumé) should be preceded by a large dot or bullet in a list format. This style makes it easy for the eyes to scan, and it effectively showcases what you want the reader to focus on. Be sure to use a bullet point instead of a diamond, arrow, star, asterisk, or other symbol. List one accomplishment or responsibility per bullet. The narrative for each bullet should ideally be on one to two lines maximum. If it gets longer than that, it becomes laborious to read. Edit to reduce the phrases and sentence(s) as needed.

Make it Lively

Start each bullet point with an action verb for an upbeat, active tone (see pages 116 to117). In other words, rather than preceding each statement with "Responsible for" or "Involved in," use more proactive language such as: Initiated, Directed, Oversaw. Example: The item, "Responsible for orientation of new hires," reads better as, "Oriented and trained new hires." You're not claiming to be the only one who does this; you're simply describing your activities in a more assertive, action-oriented way.

Brevity is Key

Use short, truncated sentences rather than complete sentences. By eliminating unnecessary words and phrases, you assist the reader in focusing in on what is important and significant. Examples —

*   **Too wordy:** *Administered primary nurse case management in home care setting to adults by assessing, developing, implementing, and evaluating each patient's plan of care.*

    More concise: Conducted adult case management in home care setting.

*   **Too wordy:** *Coordinated all aspects of clinical drug study, including data collection, accurate maintenance of records according to study protocol, completion of case report forms, and interaction with physicians.*

    More concise: Coordinated all aspects of clinical drug studies.

Use Clear Headings

Create category headings (Experience, Education, etc.) in upper case letters and in bold print so they are easy to spot. Position all headings in the same place throughout the document, either in the center of the page or to the far left (flush left). This way the readers can quickly find what they're looking for.

Be Clear and Specific

Keep the language simple and clear throughout. Avoid vague and generalized statements such as: "Initiate care of plan with recommendations to physicians and provide ongoing progress assessments" or "Another facet of my position is to interface with physicians and all staff members to allow the patient a positive perioperative experience." Not only are both of these statements vague, they relate to very basic, routine duties, which do not belong on your résumé. Here's an example of a confusing statement: "Utilized dynamic, interpersonal, and negotiation talents to develop and maintain cohesive relationships with hospital discharge planners, thereby substantially expanding and diversifying the source of temporary employment vacancies from supplemental positions within hospitals to home care opportunities."

Interestingly enough, this statement appeared on a functional résumé under the heading of "Communication Skills." Not only is the sentence wordy and complex, but the reader would be hard-pressed to understand its meaning. I was exhausted just reading it.

Résumé Content

Later in this chapter (How to Develop and Update your Résumé), we'll discuss how to gather the information needed to start developing your résumé content. Right now, we'll discuss how to choose that which is most important and interesting in your background and how to present it in the best possible light. Here are some general guidelines for developing content.

Be Selective

When choosing what to include on your résumé, less is more. Everyone is on information overload these days so you don't need to mention everything you've ever done. When describing work experiences, avoid routine duties and focus on that which is most important and interesting.

Expand Your Vision

Show a diversity of experience (see Skills/Experience inventory chart); don't focus on clinical skills alone as that is only one aspect of what a nurse does. Include any speaking or writing you did, business or managerial experience acquired, special projects worked on, interdisciplinary committees you sat on, etc. If you are a new nurse or worked off-shifts or per diem and therefore have had limited experiences, at least enhance or "punch up" the description of your clinical skills. Examples: "IV certified, Proficient in ventilator management, Conducted patient and family teaching," sounds much better than: "Picked up doctor's orders, Delivered patient meds, Took vital signs." Your résumé should not read like a job description.

Spell it Out

Don't use undefined acronyms, making your résumé a sea of alphabet soup. Remember, many people in other specialties may not know the acronyms common in your specialty. Even if you are applying for a job in the same specialty you currently work in, human resource (HR) professionals will likely be reading and screening your résumé before it gets to someone in your specialty. If the HR people can't understand it, they may disregard it. The general rule when using an acronym is to spell it out the first time you use it. Example: "Cardiac Step-Down Unit (CSDU)." After that, you can use the acronym throughout the document.

Show Progression of Responsibility

Demonstrate an increase in responsibility and position when possible. For example, if you were originally hired as a staff nurse and later promoted to charge nurse, rather than listing both positions separately list it once as:

- Hired as staff nurse. After two years, promoted to shift supervisor. One year later, promoted to nurse manager.

Then, proceed to list bullet points of information related to your highest level of authority. Of course, you can include significant experiences or accomplishments from your original positions, too, as long as you don't overdo it.

Focus on the Here and Now

The older the position is, the less you need to say about it. Your résumé should focus on the most recent and most important information. (See FAQ section of this chapter about how far back to go on your résumé.)

Pump it Up with Numbers

Use quantitative data (numbers or percentages) whenever possible to demonstrate scope of responsibility, especially in supervisory and administrative roles such as:

- Dollar amount of the budget you managed
- Number and type of staff you were responsible for
- Size of unit or facility worked in (number of beds, volume of outpatient visits per year)
- What your sales volume was

Show Results

Use quantitative data as applicable to demonstrate results achieved, such as:

- Percentage of decrease of undesirable outcomes, such as infections, falls, or staff turnover attributable to special projects/policies you developed or implemented
- Percentage of increase of desirable results, such as increased sales volume

Don't Repeat Yourself

If you did essentially the same thing at more than one place of employment, don't list identical bullet points of information under both jobs. That is boring and redundant. Try to vary the wording and the description if possible.

Key Elements

Organize your résumé in a way that makes it easy for the reader to quickly find whatever information he or she is looking for. It should be broken down into general categories and should contain certain basic information. Following is information about how to maximize each section of your résumé so the information works to your best advantage.

Identifying Information

At the top of the first page of your résumé, include your name, address, and phone number. Also include your cell phone number and e-mail address if you have one. Fax number is optional. You can put some initials after your name if you wish, such as: Kurt Allen, RN, BA. However, it is not necessary to include all of your credentials here. You can enumerate those in the Education and Certification sections of your résumé. At the top of subsequent pages, it is only necessary to include your name and page number. Suggestion: Put your name in bold print to make it stand out.

Objective vs. Summary

Contrary to what you may have heard, it is not necessary to include an objective on your résumé. In fact, an objective can actually work against you. Here's why.

Most people use one of two types of objectives. The first is position-specific, such as "Looking for a position in case management." The problem with this is that if you apply for another type of position, you will have to redo your résumé to amend or remove that statement. This is not practical or always even possible because of time constraints. Besides, if you're applying for a case management job, it should be fairly obvious that your objective is to find a position in case management. And, since a cover letter would normally accompany a résumé that is mailed, faxed, or e-mailed, that would be the place to mention which specific position you are applying for or what your areas of interest are.

The other type of objective consists of a flowery statement that says something general like: "Looking for a position where I can utilize all of my skills and abilities to deliver excellent patient care." This statement is vague, general, and virtually meaningless. So what's the point? Remember that you have only three seconds to 20 seconds to grab the interest and attention of the reader. And since the first few lines on your résumé are the first thing the reader is likely to look at, you want it to be strong, energizing, and interesting. Note: If attending a career fair or facility open house where a cover letter is not customarily used, you can mention to the recruiter if you have a particular preference of position or department.

A good alternative to the objective is the Summary. I am not referring to a summary of qualifications that some people use where they list, in summary form, what's already in their résumé. Rather I am referring to a short paragraph made up of two to three powerful, punchy sentences that represent the best you have to offer. The first sentence should give an overview of your experience. The second and third sentence should convey strong personality traits, one or two exceptional skills or abilities, and other desirable attributes.

Here are a few examples:

- RN with unique background combining both healthcare and business experience. Possess excellent teaching and training skills. Detail-oriented, energetic, and creative problem solver.

- New graduate nurse brimming with enthusiasm and drive. Possess a good work ethic and a strong desire to be a successful professional nurse. Have developed excellent communication skills and am not afraid to ask questions or ask for help as needed.

- LPN with more than 25 years of diverse experience in acute care, long-term care, and community health. Conscientious clinician who loves direct patient care as much as supervision and training. Considered a team player and self-starter.

- Seasoned administrator with a proven record of streamlining inefficient operations and creating profitable departments. Well versed in regulatory affairs. Considered approachable, fair-minded, and results-oriented.

- Experienced nurse educator who is passionate about teaching. Accomplished writer, speaker, and trainer. Creative, high-energy, and very organized professional with a great sense of humor.

This type of summary serves as an introduction to you. The examples above are high-energy and grab the reader's attention. They draw the reader in, provide a good feeling about the candidate, and make him or her want to read more...and hopefully learn more about you by bringing you in for an interview. And while some may criticize the use of clichés such as "Team-player" and "Self-starter," the truth is that these phrases are still commonly used by employers and recruiters in classified ads, job descriptions, and interviews and elicit a positive response from them.

Employer Information

List the employer's name followed by city and state. It is not necessary to include a complete address for each employer on your résumé. If a prospective employer wants that information, they'll ask you to provide it on an application or reference form. It is a good idea to put the employer's name in bold print so that it stands out.

Your Title

List your current or last title held under the employer's name followed by the department(s) or unit(s) if applicable. Consider putting your title in italics to make it stand out and to differentiate it from the rest of the print.

If you were a staff nurse or unit manager on more than one unit but with similar responsibilities, you can list the title once, followed by the units.

Example: *Staff Nurse, Orthopedics, Medical/Surgical, Telemetry*

If you've had several different titles/positions over the years with the same employer, other than promotions within the same department, list other titles separately. In this case, list the employer's name only once with total years of employment there. When listing each position, put the years associated with it in parenthesis next to the title.

Example:

Country Side Medical Center, Calico, NY   **1990-2000**
Unit Manager, Psychiatry (1998-2000)

Include a position overview (see below) and several bullet points as appropriate. Repeat this method with subsequent titles at the same place of employment.

Position Overview

If using a chronological résumé, under each position listed in the "Experience" section, give a one-sentence overview that conveys the scope of responsibility or a general description of the type of work you did (see example #1).

Employment Dates

List dates of employment either to the right of the employer's name or to the left; either way is correct. However, listing them to the right of the page is preferable for several reasons. Since we read from left to right, our eyes automatically scan the left side of the page first. Therefore, listing dates of employment on the right forces the reader to focus on your experience and accomplishments rather than your dates of employment.

It is not necessary to use an exact date of employment start and stop (month and day), but only the year. For example, if you worked somewhere from January 3, 2002, to August 4, 2005, you only need to state "2002-2005." If you worked from January to December of 1999, just put "1999." This can help to smooth out some rough edges on your résumé if you have trouble spots with your dates. Besides, employers don't want or need that much information on your résumé.

Note: Don't confuse filling out a job application with developing a professional résumé. They are two entirely different documents. If an employer asks you to fill out an application, which requires the month of employment start and stop, then you can provide that information on the application. However, since every employer is different, when asked to fill out a job application, ask, "Can I just attach my résumé?" If they ask you to also fill out the application, ask if you need to complete the whole thing or just certain parts. Since both documents are used in different ways, comply with their request.

Note: Once you become self-employed or if you are working as a consultant, you can eliminate the dates of employment on a functional résumé.

Categories

In addition to Work Experience, traditional résumé categories include: Education, Licenses and Certifications, Special Skills, Professional Affiliations, and Community/Volunteer Work, not necessarily in that order. Additional categories, such as Awards and Honors, Publications, Presentations, and Military Service, may be used if applicable. Following are some guidelines for each.

Licenses and Certifications

List all professional licenses you carry in any state. For example, if you are applying for a job in Maryland and hold Maryland and California nursing licenses, list them both. It is not necessary to list your actual nursing license number or year of issue or expiration on your résumé.

Only list current information; no one is interested in what certifications or licenses you've had in the past if they have lapsed for reasons other than disciplinary actions. It is also not necessary to list the date you first became certified in something. Too many irrelevant details clog up your résumé.

Remember to spell out certification acronyms. Example: Certified Operating Room Nurse (CNOR). If you only list the acronym, and the reader doesn't know what it stands for, you might as well leave it off your résumé for all the good it will do. You may want to include the organization that issued the certification, but this is optional.

Education

List your highest level of education first and work your way down from there. If you are currently enrolled in school for a higher degree, put that first to highlight that you are pursuing a higher degree as follows:

City College
Master's degree in nursing — currently pursuing

Be sure to include all of your degrees, including nonnursing degrees.

If you took a certain number of credits at a college, but never finished the degree and are not currently active in the program, you can state it this way:

City College 32 graduate level credits completed

Of course, it is advisable to enroll in even one course so that you can say "Currently pursuing" as above and work toward completion.

If you started your degree program in one school and finished it up in another, it is only necessary to list the school that issued your diploma.

There is no need to note the start date of any educational experience. There is also no need to include the date you graduated from any educational program unless you are a new graduate nurse. Likewise, it is not necessary to include anticipated graduation dates for education unless you are a student nurse in a basic nursing education program. This does not apply to licensed nurses who are advancing their education. (See Special Situations.)

If you received school-related honors or special recognition such as cum laude or other academic awards, you should include them. However, it is not necessary to include a list of academic scholarships.

High school information generally is not included on a professional résumé with a few exceptions. If you had outstanding or unusual achievements demonstrating leadership, community service, or notable academic accomplishments, you might consider adding them. I once coached a nurse who had a swimming scholarship named after her in high school because of her leadership abilities. That is an honor worth noting and makes a very positive statement about the nurse. Therefore, we decided to include this information on her résumé under Awards/Honors.

If you are a new graduate nurse and attended nursing school right out of high school, it could be beneficial to initially include select information from high school years on your résumé, such as being a member or officer of a Future Nurses of America Club, or if you were a member of a healthcare association, such as Health Occupations Students of America (HOSA). However, once you cease to be a new graduate nurse (one to two years after graduation, regardless of experience), this type of information is no longer relevant and should be removed from your résumé.

It is not advisable to list continuing education (CE) credits here. That's because a laundry list of CE courses taken only serves to clutter up your résumé. Employers are primarily concerned with your formal education and degrees. You can mention any relevant CE courses in your cover letter or on an interview. If you really want to, you can write something here, such as Continuing Education Courses/Credits available upon request, to indicate that you have taken them. However, this is not necessary.

Special Skills

This is the place to highlight special skills and abilities, beyond that which is already on your résumé, such as basic and advanced computer skills, languages spoken and written, good writing and speaking skills, etc.

Awards and Honors

List special recognition you have received from employers, professional associations, or your community, including attendance awards, nurse of the year, service awards, etc. As an alternative, employment related awards can be listed as a bullet point under a specific job.

Professional Affiliations

List professional associations you currently belong to. Spell out the name of the organizations listed. There is no need to include the date you joined the organization. It is not necessary to list offices held in the past unless you are a past president. Be selective about including current leadership positions held as well as special projects and committees worked on. If you have other professional association experience, past or present, that is relevant to a job you are applying for, you can mention that in your cover letter. For example, if you are applying for a job in education, you can mention in your cover letter that you were active on the education committee of an association and elaborate on the types of things you did that are relevant to this position.

When listing an organization whose name is not self-explanatory, such as Sigma Theta Tau International, it is advisable to add an explanatory phrase such as "Honor society for nursing" since many people, including other nurses, do not know what STTI is. Remember, if the reader doesn't know what something is or what it means, then the information is meaningless.

Publications

If you have published work, by all means list that. This would include articles published online or in print publications, chapters written for books, etc. If you have only one or two published works, list them under the heading Publications. If you have more than a few, it's best to use the heading Selected Publications. This implies that what you have listed is a sampling of what you've written but that there is more. List only a few of the most recent or more significant works under this heading. A full listing, along with a writing sample, can always be submitted separately if requested. It is not necessary to list these publications in full bibliography format on a résumé. (See résumé example #2.)

Presentations

If you have done a few major presentations at conferences, conventions, and career fairs, list them under the heading Presentations. As with publications, use Selected Presentations, if the list is longer.

Presentations might be listed in this way:

Managing the Patient with Type I Diabetes. Arkansas Nurses Association Annual Convention 2005.

Presentations done as part of one's employment can be included in summary form as a bullet point under that place of employment.

Example:

- Present regularly at inservice sessions, new employee orientation, and community outreach programs on topics such as management of diabetes, foot care, and nutrition.

Volunteer/Community Work

Be selective but do include those activities, both past and present that demonstrate leadership and other important and relevant skills and experiences as well as civic involvement. Be sure to include all healthcare-related volunteer experience and work with youth groups, the elderly, the homeless, etc. Be cautious in listing work with organizations that would reveal your religious or political affiliations such as the Young Republican Club or Right-to-Life group. Aside from being personal and protected, this type of information can work against you.

Military Service

List the type of duty you did (active or reserves), the branch of the service, your rank, and the type of work you did. Include any special commendations or medals.

What *Not* to Put on Your Résumé

When it comes to your résumé, some things are best left unsaid. Unnecessary and inappropriate information can make you look unsophisticated and unprofessional. It can also serve to distract the reader from your accomplishments and more important information. Here are several examples of things best left off your résumé.

Don't list hobbies like sewing, reading, or skiing. While a few prospective employers may claim this gives them insight into your personality, most recruiters find it too folksy and even irksome. Exception: Some activities can reflect positively on you, such as having formerly competed in a particular sport, running a marathon, and winning related awards even on a local level. These might be listed on your résumé under Additional Information or Other Accomplishments or mentioned in your cover letter.

Don't list personal information, such as health status, height, and weight. This has no place on your professional résumé.

Don't list your age or martial status. This is protected information under current employment laws.

Don't list where or when you went to high school. It is considered irrelevant. However, there are exceptions to every rule. If, for example, you are a fairly new nurse, and you attended a vocational or technical high school where you were trained as a nurse's aide or other caregiver, then it would be appropriate to list that education (see Education section above) at least until you've accumulated significant graduate nurse experience.

Don't list any salary information on your résumé. We'll get into this subject more in-depth in subsequent chapters, but suffice it to say it doesn't belong on your résumé.

Don't write "References available upon request" at the bottom of your résumé or list actual references with contact information in the body of your résumé. It is understood that if an employer wants references, they will ask for them, and you will supply them. Otherwise, you don't get the job. End of story. The point is that you want to eliminate everything that is unnecessary from your résumé. You want to declutter it.

Don't type the word, Résumé, on the top of the document. (I've seen this more times than I can count.) If the prospective employer can't figure out that it's a résumé by looking at it, then you have more serious problems!

Appearance

First impressions are important in your personal appearance and so too in your résumé. That is why your résumé must be picture perfect. Its overall look will make an impression before the reader even reads one word. Here's what you need to know.

Paper

Use good quality 8 $\frac{1}{2}$ x 11 bond paper. Bond paper has high cotton fiber content and is used for stationary, as opposed to copy machine or computer paper. Choose a paper that looks and feels good. It should be 20 lb. weight (denotes the thickness and body of the paper) and have a watermark (an embedded logo visible when held up the light). Either linen or a flat finish (surface) is appropriate. Ask your local printer to show you some samples of good quality résumé paper. Be cautious of boxed paper labeled "résumé paper" in some office supply chains. Often this is lower-grade, coarse paper and not professional in look or feel.

Color

Stick to white or off-white paper. Although grey or cream color is generally considered acceptable, it can appear muddy when the document is faxed, photocopied, or electronically scanned (passed through a machine for storage on computer disc).

Print

Only use black ink. Black print on white paper creates the best contrast for easy readability and makes a very professional looking document. The print quality must be crisp, dark, sharp, and clear. Therefore, every copy of your résumé should be individually printed on a letter-quality laser printer — not photocopied. If you do not have such a printer, have your résumé printed by someone who does or bring it on disc to your local print shop or stationary store for printing. If the print on your résumé is fuzzy, light, or of otherwise poor quality, it will be difficult to read and may be disregarded and discarded. Print only on one side of the paper.

Character Size and Style

The type size (size of the letters) should be 12 point. Anything smaller is difficult to read. If the recruiter can't read it, it may wind up in the trash. And, since many employers electronically scan résumés for storage on computer discs, 12-point type is preferable for scanning. Stick with an easily readable font (character style), such as Times New Roman.

Length

Résumés should be one to two pages in length on average. There is a common myth that nursing résumés should be on one page, but that has never been the case. By the time you list even one job along with your education and credentials, you're already on two pages, which is perfectly acceptable. On rare occasions, I would recommend a three-page résumé for someone with exceptional and extensive experience and credentials, but that would be the exception rather than the rule. Remember, less is more when it comes to résumé writing.

Margins

Margins should be approximately one-inch on the top, bottom, and sides of each page of your résumé. You can alter those dimensions slightly, if necessary, but don't get carried away. If you need a bit more space on the page, it is better to reduce the top and bottom margins rather than the side margins. The empty space beyond the margins and anywhere that there is no printing is known as "white space." White space makes the printed part of the sheet easier to read and comprehend.

Some additional tips:

- Keep all information about one employer on the same page if possible. In other words, if you list a particular employer toward the bottom of the first page, try to list all information related to that employment on

I once saw a résumé where the print literally took up the entire surface on the page. There were no margins at all. This nurse had heard that your résumé should be on one page, so figured if he eliminated the margins, he could cram more information on one page. This is simply not acceptable. Not only is a document without margins difficult to follow, but it is completely unprofessional.

that page rather than continuing it on the second page. The exception would be if you held multiple positions/titles in that place of employment and simply can't fit it all on the first page. In that case, you could list the employer's name again at the top of the second page followed by "(continued)" and start with a new position held at that place of employment. In other words, don't split information about one employer, or at least not about one job title, onto two pages, if you can help it.

- Stay away from fancy borders, designs, clip-art, or background images on your résumé, such as shooting stars, flowers, clouds, or a caduceus. (I've seen all of these.) There is no place for this on a professional résumé, and it only serves to distract the reader.

- Don't staple or tape the pages of your résumé together.

Special Situations

There are some situations that require special handling. Here are several examples of unique situations and ways to focus on the positive and minimize the negative.

The Mature Nurse

Age discrimination is alive and well in the world we live in. Fortunately, it is at a minimum in nursing. However, it is still wise to keep your résumé age-neutral as much as possible. There are several ways to shift the reader's attention to your experience by eliminating information that would make it obvious how old or young you likely are. For example, if you list your first job as starting in 1960, or note that you graduated from nursing school or other post-secondary school that year, it is inevitable that the reader will mentally calculate your approximate age.

One way to minimize the age factor is to only go back 15 years to 20 years with your employment history as outlined in the Q&A section on page 111. It is also advisable not to list the actual dates that you graduated from any educational programs. The exception, as noted in the Education section above, is if you are a new graduate nurse regardless of your chronological age. (Today's new graduate nurses range from 20 years to 70 years of age.)

The New Graduate Nurse

The big question is whether to list information related to major student clinical rotations on your résumé. If you are a new graduate who came to nursing school with little or no prior work experience, then the listing of clinical rotations on your résumé can provide relevant content. Just be sure to correctly categorize this experience as Student Clinical Rotations rather than Work Experience. Recruiters are interested to see what types of facilities you did those rotations in (teaching hospital vs. community hospital). They are also interested to see if you did any of your rotations in a facility within their healthcare system.

If you have some prior healthcare work experience (worked as a nurses aide, practical nurse, respiratory therapist, etc.), then it is generally not necessary to include content related to student clinical rotations. However, you can mention related information in your cover letter that might be of interest to a recruiter, such as the information mentioned in the above paragraph.

If you went to nursing school right out of high school, include work experience you had before or during nursing school, especially those positions pertinent to dealing with people, like waitress or sales clerk.

If you are a recent nursing school graduate (within the last two years), you should include your date of graduation from nursing school so that your status is clear.

It is not necessary, nor advisable, to list your grade point average (GPA) on your résumé. Although you will hear some varying opinions about this, the vast majority of recruiters agree that GPA is not an indictor of a good clinical nurse and do not put much stock in it. Also, the information can unwittingly work against you if it is less than a 4.0. For example, a recruiter may be reviewing multiple résumés, several of which have included GPAs. The fact that one nurse has a higher or lower GPA than another can subconsciously impact the recruiter one way or the other, and you will find that it is not always in the way you would think.

If someone is interested in knowing what your GPA is, they will ask for it, and you can provide it. If you do opt to list it on your résumé for some reason, eliminate it once you are out of school for a year or more as it will no longer be relevant.

The Student Nurse

If you are a student nurse, you should include your anticipated date of graduation in the Education section of your résumé. That gives a prospective employer some idea of when you will be eligible for licensure. You can also list student clinical rotations completed to date, as a new graduate nurse would.

How to Develop and Update Your Résumé

Now that you've reviewed résumé writing basics, it's time to put what you've learned into action. The process of developing a good résumé may seem daunting, especially the first time you try to do it, but the effort will be well worth it. Once done, you only need to revise and update it periodically, a much easier task then creating it from scratch. Here are steps to take to create or revamp your résumé.

Step 1. Gather Pertinent Information

Do some preliminary work by recording basic information about your education, licenses and certifications, and other key résumé elements. Make a list of all employers you've had, dates of employment, and title(s) held.

Step 2. Write It All Down

Create one work sheet for each employer/position and jot down everything you can think of that you did while employed there. This is a preliminary phase, so record it all. You can weed through it later. Do the same for professional association involvement and volunteer/community work if applicable. Once you've done all of this, put the information aside and go back to it several times over the next few days to add information as it comes to you. It will take some time to recall everything.

• •

When I was developing my first professional résumé years ago, I drafted something based on my recollection of what I had done in each position I'd had up until then. For the position at the medical weight-control center, I had listed some basic things related to my day-to-day responsibilities. I asked my husband to look it over and tell me what he thought. Related to that position, he said, "What about the fact that you opened a new center for them, researched the demographics, oversaw renovations on the space, hired and trained all the staff, and built the business up?" I was startled when I heard him say it that way because, not only had I actually forgotten about all that, it sounded so impressive when he said it! Sometimes we need input from others to appreciate how much we do.

• •

Step 3. Seek Input from Others

It's a good idea to ask a spouse, coworker, supervisor or friend to help you remember some of the more significant things you did while in a particular job. We are notorious for forgetting, overlooking, and minimizing things that we've done!

Step 4. Choose a Format and Lay It Out

Once you have gathered the pertinent information and feel you have developed a comprehensive listing of accomplishments and experiences, choose the résumé format that is best for you. Start to lay out your résumé according to the samples at the end of this chapter. Choose information from your worksheets that is most appropriate and significant (Review Résumé Content section starting on page 94). Break the information down into sound bites or bullet points so that each conveys only one accomplishment, responsibility, or piece of information.

Step 5. Craft the Wording

Now start to work on the wording of the information after each bullet point. Choose an action verb to begin each statement when possible. Truncate and shorten the statements so that each word has impact. Remember: Each bullet point should be one sentence/statement and ideally on one or two lines maximum. If it gets longer than that, you probably need to edit it down. (Review Lay-Out and Writing Style section.) Ask yourself: Can I say it better? Can I say it in a more powerful, proactive way? Can I be more concise? Can I be clearer?

Step 6. Let it Rest, Then Edit

Once you've done this, set it aside for a day or so if possible. When you come back to it, do more editing. Eliminate anything that is routine, redundant, irrelevant, old, or uninteresting. Repeat this process until you are satisfied with the content and the wording. It is common to do several edits

"I update my résumé as soon as I start a job and include the new position, so my résumé is updated and ready to go at a moment's notice."

— Experienced Nurse Agnes

before coming up with a final draft. Think of a good cook boiling down the juices and broth to make a rich sauce.

Step 7. Go Over It with a Fine-Toothed Comb

Look your résumé over for consistent layout and to check for spelling, grammar, and punctuation errors. Have one or two other people do the same. It is very easy to miss errors on a document you have looked at repeatedly. Remember, your résumé has to be picture perfect. Don't rely on the spell check and grammar feature on your computer. It is also good to have someone else look it over to make sure it is clear, concise, and complete.

Frequently Asked Questions

Q: *Should I tailor my résumé to fit each job I apply for?*

A: No. That is not practical or necessary. For the most part, you should be able to develop one good, comprehensive résumé that will be applicable to most situations. Your cover letter is the place to customize; here you can mention specific elements of your background that relate to a particular position. (See Chapter 6.)

Q: *What if I work for a staffing or travel nurse agency — should I list every hospital I've worked at?*

A: No. Since you were not an employee of any of the hospitals, you would simply list the name of the agency you worked for. And since some nurses work for more than one agency at a time, it is not even necessary to list each agency. Rather, in place of an employer's name, use the generic title Travel Nurse or Agency Nurse. (See example #1.)

Q: *What if I've worked for two or more employers at the same time — how do I list that?*

A: Simply list all positions as you would any others, listing the most significant one first. The résumé reader will likely note the date overlap. Many nurses have had more than one position at a time, myself included, so this is not unusual. A past employer told me that this was one of the reasons why he hired me for a management position. He figured that if I could juggle two jobs at one time I could probably handle anything that came my way.

Q: *How far back should I go in listing my experience?*

A: There is no hard and fast rule here. Most prospective employers agree that they are only interested in the last 15 years to 20 years of steady employment history. That does not mean that you should *only* list employment back to that point. Besides, some people have been at the same place of employment for longer for that! Do go back a reasonable period of time, realizing that things you did more than 20 years ago have minimal relevance. If you had significant work experience prior to that, which is different from what you have done in the last 15 years to 20 years, you could add an explanatory sentence at the end of your Work Experience section. For example, if you have worked primarily in education or nontraditional positions for the last 20 years, and want to indicate that you have a solid clinical foundation, you could add a sentence at the end of the section such as, "Prior to this, had significant clinical experience in several major medical centers."

If your last 15 years to 20 years of employment have been primarily clinical, it is not necessary to add that additional statement. If you have older work experience that is directly related to a job you are applying for, you can mention that in your cover letter.

Note: If you have been out of the workforce for a significant period of time (seven to eight or more years), list your last several jobs, even if they were more than 10 years to 15 years ago, to show some employment history.

Q: *Should I include nonnursing work experience?*

A: Definitely! Years ago, nurses were told not to include other work experience on their résumé. However, that has changed. Nursing, and nurses themselves, are more diverse than ever today. Many individuals are coming into nursing as a second and third career and that prior work experience is both interesting and relevant.

Q: *Do I have to list every job, even the ones I stayed at for a few weeks or months? In other words, is it OK to eliminate some things?*

A: That depends on how long you were at a particular job and why you left. If you had a job for a very short period of time, say a few weeks, and left because the job wasn't a good fit for you, you might opt not to include that on your résumé. If you left a job for any reason during an orientation period, you do not necessarily need to list that since employment is generally considered "conditional" during that time. If you were at a job for several months or more, then it becomes risky to eliminate it. Not only will there appear to be a gap in your employment history (unless you had another job at the same time), but also there is more likelihood that your prospective employer will uncover this information through networking and reference checking. Use your judgment, but be cautious.

A word of caution: Some states have laws requiring full disclosure by licensed healthcare workers of past employment. These laws exist to facilitate a thorough background check and to protect the public. However, these laws apply more to an employment application, which is an official document, rather than to your résumé, which is a personal document.

Q: *Should the education section be listed before or after my work experience? I've seen it done both ways.*

A: Either way is correct. However, a traditional résumé usually includes the education category after work experience. The curriculum vitae would list education at the beginning of the document after the summary if one were used. (See Chapter 6.)

Q: *Do you recommend using a résumé writing service?*

A: I don't, for several reasons. Just because someone provides résumé writing services, doesn't mean they necessarily produce effective résumés. Anyone with some computer skills can produce the document but that does not mean that they know how to maximize your experiences on paper or even that they are up on current résumé writing standards. Many of these résumés have a vaguely generic quality to them and are often referred to as "canned résumés" by professional résumé readers. In other words, they have a certain "formula" look and feel to them. This is a turn-off to a recruiter or prospective employer. I have seen too many bland, boring, and ineffective nursing résumés written by so-called "Résumé Writers" who list nothing more than routine nursing duties in an outdated format. The only person who benefits from this is the résumé writer.

While résumé writing is intimidating to most, once you learn how to do it and take the time and make the effort to develop one, you empower yourself on many levels. No one will develop a better résumé for you than you yourself can. And, once you have a good basic résumé, keeping it updated is easy. I have worked with hundreds of nurses over the years to assist them in developing a powerful résumé for themselves. I frequently heard, "It wasn't as hard as I thought it would be once I sat down to do it."

That being said, I realize that some people will still want or need the help of another person with résumé development and writing. In that case, it would be ideal to work with a nursing career coach or career counselor familiar with the scope of what nurses do, as well as one who is up on current résumé writing standards.

Q: *If I worked part time or per diem, do I have to note that?*

A: No. List the position as usual, but it is not necessary to mention your status on your résumé. You can mention it if it comes up in conversation, or if you are asked.

Q: *If I've been out of the work force for awhile, how do I indicate that, or account for my time on my résumé?*

A: You don't. You can address that in your cover letter. (See Chapter 6.)

Q: *I'm confused; why is there so much differing information out there about what should and shouldn't be on a résumé?*

A: There are several reasons for that. Some people who casually dole out career advice are regurgitating outdated information based on what they've seen and heard or what they believe to be true. They are often not career management specialists and have done no research or have no actual career management experience to draw from. They are also not in touch with those who actually hire and promote. Always consider the source when getting career advice.

Another reason is that there are some differing opinions and preferences about certain résumé details. For example, some recruiters might advise that you include an objective on your résumé because that is what they are accustomed to or what they prefer. However, most will tell you that it is neither necessary nor advisable for the reasons I have stated. The information and advice in this book is a synopsis of what the vast majority of career management experts, recruiters, and prospective employers have to say about career development, including résumé writing.

We'll continue our discussion of résumés and CVs in Chapter 6.

Most Common Faults Observed by Résumé Readers

- Poor overall appearance (paper, print, layout)
- Misspellings, bad grammar, poor punctuation
- Not mentioning accomplishments
- Print too small
- Too wordy
- Too long
- Too short, sparse (no detail provided, lacks content)
- Mentioning personal and other irrelevant information
- Lengthy and complex sentences, paragraphs, phrases
- Difficult to comprehend, decipher (too many acronyms, unclear language)
- Key category/information missing (e.g. education, licenses and certifications, etc.)

Résumé Skills/Experience Inventory

This list is provided to remind you of your own experiences and to help you focus in on the type of specific experiences and accomplishments that should be listed on a résumé. These are only examples and constitute a partial list. There are many others.

Speaking & Teaching

Presenting at grand rounds
Developing and presenting in-services
Providing patient and family teaching and counseling
Conducting community education
Acting as preceptor/mentor to new hires, new graduates
Working with students
Development of teaching aides (brochures, booklets, videos)

Business and Managerial

Taking occasional charge or supervision
Promotions you received
Working on the budget or schedule
Involvement with special projects such as developing or updating policies and procedures, research, quality improvement
Manuals or special forms developed
Being part of new programs implemented
Liaison with outside agencies
Special committee/project work related to department start-up, reengineering, cost-cutting, reorganizing, installation of new computer system, etc.

Committee Work

Any special or standing committees that you sat on or chaired, such as discharge planning, quality improvement, recruitment and retention, safety, etc. These can be unit-specific, nursing department, or facility-wide committees.

Additional

Participating in employer-sponsored health fairs, health screenings, and recruitment events.

Clinical Skills

Any special skills (beyond the routine) that you developed proficiency in such as chemotherapy, ventilator management, ostomy and wound care, diabetic teaching, etc.

Action Verbs

Accomplished	Achieved	Acted
Adapted	Adopted	Administrated
Advanced	Advised	Arranged
Assimilated	Attained	Augmented
Authored	Built	Chaired
Coached	Collaborated	Communicated
Completed	Composed	Conceived
Conducted	Consolidated	Consulted
Contributed	Controlled	Coordinated
Counseled	Created	Decreased
Delivered	Demonstrated	Designed
Developed	Devised	Directed
Edited	Educated	Eliminated
Empowered	Enforced	Established
Exceeded	Excelled	Executed
Expedited	Facilitated	Formulated
Fostered	Founded	Furthered
Generated	Guided	Handled
Headed	Identified	Implemented
Improved	Increased	Influenced
Initiated	Innovated	Inspired
Instituted	Instructed	Integrated
Interfaced	Interviewed	Introduced

Launched	Lectured	Led
Liaised	Lowered	Maintained
Managed	Marketed	Mediated
Mentored	Met	Motivated
Negotiated	Operated	Optimized
Orchestrated	Organized	Originated
Overhauled	Oversaw	Paved
Performed	Persuaded	Piloted
Pioneered	Planned	Practiced
Prepared	Presented	Presided
Prevented	Produced	Progressed
Promoted	Proposed	Provided
Published	Ran	Reduced
Rejuvenated	Renegotiated	Reorganized
Represented	Researched	Resolved
Restored	Restructured	Revised
Revitalized	Revolutionized	Scheduled
Screened	Secured	Selected
Served as	Specialized	Started
Strategized	Streamlined	Strengthened
Structured	Succeeded	Supervised
Surpassed	Taught	Trained
Transformed	Translated	Unified
Updated	Upgraded	Wrote

Sample #1 Chronological Format

JANICE SMITH, RN, BSN

45 Lane Avenue

Smithville, New Jersey 00090

(908) 555-2222

jsmith@net.net

SUMMARY

RN with diverse clinical and managerial experience in critical care and long term care settings. Excellent training skills. Possess positive, can-do attitude. Considered a team player and self-starter.

EXPERIENCE

SMITHVILLE GENERAL HOSPITAL, Smithville, NJ   1992-Present

Clinical Manager, Telemetry Unit

Clinical and administrative responsibility for 30-bed unit, including finances, personnel, and regulatory compliance
- Hired as a staff nurse, promoted to Clinical Manager after 8 months
- Designed and implemented a quality management program for unit
- Represent Department of Nursing on the following interdisciplinary committees: Infection Control; Utilization Management
- Frequent speaker for public outreach programs
- Act as preceptor to new hires

TOWNSHIP MEMORIAL HOSPITAL, Township, NJ   1990-1991

Staff Nurse, Emergency/Out Patient Department

Responsible for all facets of triage, emergency patient care, inpatient procedures, and minor surgery
- Directed outpatient clinics
- Administrated public screening programs
- Conducted orientation for new hires
- Coordinated department in-service
- Received perfect attendance award

TRAVEL NURSE   1988-1990

Worked with various healthcare travel agencies at temporary positions across the country from Hawaii to New York
- Developed proficiency in mechanical ventilator management
- Offered full-time positions at each facility
- Adapted to diverse work assignments including burn, oncology and pediatric units
- Assimilated easily, interpersonally, into each facility

©Donna Cardillo. Reprinted with permission.

JANICE SMITH   Page 2

UPSTATE LONG TERM CARE CENTER, Upstate, NJ   1983-1987
Staff Nurse, Sub-Acute Unit

Responsible for all aspects of medical, rehabilitative and psychosocial needs of patient
- Assumed weekend charge position
- Supervised nurses aides and LPNs
- Proficient in EKG's and venipuncture
- Co-authored department policy and procedure manual

STATE HOSPITAL, Inner City, New Jersey   1981-1983
Staff Nurse, Medical/Surgical Unit

EDUCATION
Mytown University, Somewhere, New Jersey
Currently pursuing Master of Science, Psychology

County College, County, New Jersey
Bachelor of Science Degree, Healthcare Management

Township Memorial Hospital School of Nursing, Township, New Jersey
Diploma, Nursing

LICENSES / CERTIFICATIONS
Licensed as Registered Nurse in New Jersey
Advanced Cardiac Life Support (ACLS), American Heart Association

PROFESSIONAL AFFILIATIONS
New Jersey State Nurses Association
American Nurses Association
Emergency Nurses Association
    Chair, Education Committee
Sigma Theta Tau International *Honor Society of Nursing*

AWARDS
MORE Award, North Carolina Nurses Association, Region 12
    For outstanding contributions and exemplary leadership

SPECIAL SKILLS
Fluent in German (speak, write, read), conversational in Spanish
Proficient in Word, Power Point, and Excel

Sample #2 Functional Format

Jeanne Farrell, RN, MA
100 Meadowlands Parkway
Faraway, NC 00911
555-980-2386
jfrn@net.net

RN with over 20 years of diverse experience in healthcare management, quality improvement, nursing education, and regulatory affairs. Dynamic speaker and trainer. Possess excellent ability to motivate, facilitate, and organize.

SPECIAL SKILLS

Speaking
Frequent workshop presenter at nursing and healthcare conferences, professional association meetings, and community groups on quality of care and regulatory issues

Teaching / Training
Trainer for ongoing employee/client relations program
Taught gerontology certification course for local community college
Volunteer lecturer for American Heart Association
Provided customized educational services for long term care facilities to enhance operations

Writing
Author of numerous published articles
Created and was editor of nursing department newsletter
Conducted peer review for continuing education articles and books

Management
Broad management experience in acute, sub-acute, and long-term care settings
Key team member in development of cardiac rehabilitative program
Managed operating budgets up to $8 million

SELECTED ACCOMPLISHMENTS

- Featured speaker in The Joint Commission teleconference on revised long-term care standards
- Developed and implemented critical pathways for acute, sub-acute, and long-term care cases
- Created medical by-laws and updated physician credentialing process
- Revised physical restraint assessment program resulting in 15% decreased utilization
- Member of Magnet Steering Committee resulting in Magnet Award
- Received commendation status from The Joint Commission and orchestrated numerous deficiency-free Department of Health (DOH) surveys in both acute and long term care settings

WORK EXPERIENCE

UNIVERSITY MEDICAL CENTER, Nursing Quality Improvement Coordinator ...1990-1996
GGM CONSULTING, Healthcare Consultant 1994-1996
CITY COLLEGE, Instructor, Business and Community Development 1994
SUNNY SIDE NURSING HOME, Assistant Administrator/Director of Nursing 1990-1994
COLLEGE HOSPITAL, Head Nurse, ICU 1989-1990
UPTOWN HOSPITAL MEDICAL CENTER, Staff Nurse, Telemetry and Oncology Units ..1988

EDUCATION

MA Education, Unger University, Long Branch, NJ
BS Nursing, Saint Peter's College, Englewood Cliffs, NJ

SELECTED PUBLICATIONS

"QI: Everyone's Job," Nursing Spectrum/NurseWeek Nursewire, December 2005.
"Managing in Turbulent Times," Long Term Care Journal, November 2005.

PROFESSIONAL AFFILIATIONS

National Association for Healthcare Quality
North Carolina League for Nurses
    Board of Directors
National Association Directors of Nursing Administration in Long Term Care
American Nurses Association
North Carolina Nurses Association
    Mentor to student members
    Media Ace

LICENSES AND CERTIFICATIONS

Registered Nurse License: New Jersey, North Carolina
Certified Professional in Healthcare Quality (CPHQ)   *National Assoc for Healthcare Quality*
Certified Nurse Administrator (CNA)   *American Nurses Credentialing Center*

COMMUNITY / VOLUNTEER WORK

YMCA Swim Instructor, adults and children
City Triathlon Club

Sample #3 New Graduate Résumé

Kurt Thomas, RN   P: 555-323-0000
1600 Paved Road   Cell: 555-331-9090
Inner City, CA 00502   kurt@net.net

SUMMARY: New Graduate RN with diverse clinical and work experience. Customer service oriented. Focused and motivated. Gets along well with coworkers, clients, and supervisors. Has an optimistic outlook and possesses a good sense of humor.

WORK EXPERIENCE

Inner City Hospital, Inner City, CA   2006
Emergency Department Technician
Provided wide range of nursing support services in high volume Level II trauma center

Karl's Sporting Goods, Uptown, CA   2002-2005
Retail Sales Associate
Managed in-store and telephone orders, provided customer service, and instructed customers in safe equipment use

Inner City Community Pool, Inner City, CA   2001
Life Guard

STUDENT CLINICAL ROTATIONS

Inner City Hospital ....Medical-Surgical/Oncology
Mountain Community Hospital ....Pediatrics
Center City Medical Center ....Psychiatry/Maternal Child Health
Visiting Nurse Service Inner City ....Community Health/Public Health
Veteran's Home ....Long Term Care

STUDENT EXTERNSHIP

Inner City Hospital, Inner City, CA   Summer 2006
Precepted clinical experience in medical/surgical intensive care unit

EDUCATION

California Community College, Los Angeles, CA
Associate Degree in Nursing 2007

LICENSES AND CERTIFICATIONS

California Registered Nurse License
Basic Life Support (BLS) Certification, American Heart Association

PROFESSIONAL AFFILIATIONS

Emergency Nurses Association
National Student Nurses Association

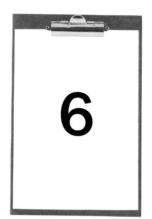

Résumé Marketing, Cover Letters, CVs, and Portfolios

lthough a traditional résumé is right for most nurses, there are certain circumstances where a curriculum vitae (CV) is more appropriate. While some folks use the terms interchangeably, a résumé and a CV are two entirely different documents and should not be confused.

A résumé, as discussed in Chapter 5, is a one- to two-page document that highlights professional accomplishments, experiences, and credentials. It is a snapshot of your career and is what most nurses need. A CV is more comprehensive, in contrast, and includes much more information and detail and is usually multiple pages long. It is generally reserved for doctoral degree-driven settings, such as higher education and original research. (Do not confuse staff nursing positions in the research department of a healthcare facility or working on clinical drug trials for a pharmaceutical company with "original research.") It may also be appropriate for high-level administrative positions or in the literary world (editor, publisher, etc.). A CV might be right for some advanced practice nurses working in the clinical setting, as well, although that is an individual decision. A CV attests to expertise and authority.

None of this is meant to automatically imply that if you have a doctoral degree or some of the above experience, you should shift to a CV. The format you use is determined more by the type of job you're applying for or the setting/specialty that you work within, rather than your credentials. Not only doesn't the average nurse need a CV, but it can be a hindrance in a normal job search by providing too much information. It is considered "overkill" in your typical job situation. However, it is a good idea to keep detailed career information for your own records. The day may come when you need to develop a CV as you transition into one of these settings. We'll discuss that in the Portfolio section later in this chapter.

Because some people use the terms CV and résumé interchangeably, when someone asks you to send your CV, it doesn't necessarily mean they want an actual CV. Unless you're applying for the type of positions mentioned above, a traditional résumé is usually what they're looking for.

Unlike a résumé, a CV does not have a set format, but certain information is customarily provided. There are also some guidelines for CVs that differ from those for a résumé. Every CV is different, so craft one that best suits your background, unique experiences, and credentials. For those of you who will be using a CV, here are some of the typical categories and components used.

CV Components

Heading

Start with a heading that includes your name, major credential acronyms, address, phone number(s), and e-mail address.

To Summarize or Not?

A summary statement, as described in Chapter 5, is optional. But since a CV is generally rather long, a summary of the candidate's particular areas of expertise and interest along with strengths and personal characteristics will be a great help to the reader.

Education

Since CVs are used in industries where higher education is both a requirement and the norm, education is traditionally listed first in the body of the document. List each school in descending order by degree starting with postgraduate work, if applicable, and going back from there. Include the degree, institution name, any honors received, major/minor, and thesis and dissertation title or description. List internships, fellowships, and similar programs.

> Although dates of education can be omitted from a traditional resume, it is customary to include them on a curriculum vitae.

With a master's thesis or doctoral dissertation, some prefer to list this as a separate category, which would include the thesis/dissertation title and provide a brief abstract (three to five sentences) discussing the content, focus, and methodology used. Including your advisor's name is optional.

Include academic achievements, such as leadership roles, grants, scholarships, awards, and recognitions as appropriate. Also mention academic affiliations, such as sororities, fraternities, societies, etc.

Professional Licenses and Certifications

Same as a résumé (See Chapter 5.)

Academic Teaching Experience

Include courses taught, courses developed and introduced, teaching interests, and a summary of teaching evaluations.

Publications/Writing

Include published works, such as journal and magazine articles, web articles, books, book chapters, and study guides. Also include work submissions and works in progress. If you have an extensive body of work, use the heading, Selected Publications, since pages and pages of publication listings lose their impact. Choose to list up to 10 to 20 published works, focusing on the most significant and recent. End with a summary statement, such as "More than 100 published articles in 60 journals. Full listing is available upon request." When a CV is too long and cumbersome, the relevant information gets lost in a sea of words, credentials, details, and paper.

Presentations

List major presentations at conferences, conventions, and symposiums, including poster presentations. If you have an extensive number of presentations, as with publications, do list a substantial number of examples, but use the phrase "Selected Presentations" and indicate the availability of a full listing upon request. There is just so much one reader can digest.

Professional Experience

It is customary to list current and past positions held along with titles and dates but not necessarily descriptions like a résumé. The format for listing employment history would be similar to a functional résumé listing.

Professional Development

This might include conferences and workshops attended.

References

Unlike a résumé, a CV might list several professional references when the candidate is looking for a new position or seeking consulting or other work. If listing references, include name, title, and contact information. These references would ideally include deans, professors, administrators, and other high-level, high-profile colleagues.

Additional Categories Might Include:

- Research/research interests
- Grants awarded
- Administrative experience
- Honors and awards
- Consulting experience
- Volunteer/Community work
- Professional association memberships and activities, including leadership roles
- Special skills, including languages spoken, and computer and technical skills

To recap, the résumé is a short summary, a snapshot of you. A CV is your portrait, your spec sheet.

Cover Letters

A well-written résumé or CV can attract the attention of prospective employers, but that's only part of the story. You also need a compelling cover letter when applying for a position or making a job inquiry. The two can be a powerful pair. In fact, some recruiters are more influenced by the cover letter than by the résumé itself. A cover letter actually speaks to the reader and helps you start the "sales" process. Here are some tips for developing a cover letter that will grab the interest of the reader and make a great first impression.

While your résumé or CV will remain somewhat static throughout a job search process, your cover letter provides an opportunity to customize your application for each position. Here is where you reveal a bit of your personality and individuality. You can also highlight specific experiences, credentials, and personal characteristics that relate to this position. And, you can mention your interest in, and familiarity with, that employer's company/facility, product, or service if applicable.

Always include a cover letter when sending a résumé or CV to a prospective employer, whether by mail, e-mail, or fax, if it is your preliminary contact with them, or if you are responding to a classified ad. The only exception would be if you were responding to an ad that specifically states, "No cover letters," or, "Send Résumé ONLY." In this case, the company is probably in a preliminary screening phase and is only interested in what credentials and recent experience a candidate does or does not have. Including a cover letter in this situation might serve to irritate and annoy the prospective employer, and you risk bumping yourself out of the running for the position before you even have a chance.

It is not necessary to send a cover letter when faxing your résumé to a headhunter or agency representative that you have just had a lengthy phone conversation with. Nor is it necessary to bring a cover letter with you to a career fair or recruitment event where you will be distributing résumés and meeting prospective employers in person.

Let's take a closer look at what goes into making a dynamite cover letter.

The Format

Create a heading at the top of your cover letter that includes your name and address. It is not necessary to list phone numbers or your e-mail address here as on a résumé.

Use a traditional business letter format that starts with the date followed by the recipient's name, title, facility, and address. If you don't have a specific person's name, address the letter to "Nurse Recruiter," "Human Resources Manager," or a department or position title mentioned in a classified ad.

Use a formal salutation, such as, "Dear Mr. Allen," or, "Dear Ms. Conrad." Ms. is the universal form of address for a woman. We discussed methods of obtaining a contact person's name in Chapter 4. If you don't have a specific person's name, you can address the letter to the entity in your address, such as, "Dear Nurse Recruiter," or, "Dear Human Resource Manager." As a last resort, you can use, "Dear Sir/Madam." Be sure to use both genders so as not to offend anyone. Avoid "To whom it may concern."

The Opening

The opening paragraph should immediately grab the reader's attention and be clear on why you are writing. If responding to a classified ad, state the position you are applying for (the company may be running multiple ads for various positions) along with the publication, and date, in which you saw the ad. You might start with something like, "I am enthusiastically applying for the Utilization Review Nurse position advertised in the *Gazette* on March 3."

If someone referred you to the person you are writing or recommended a particular position, mention that up front. Example: "Carl Howard from 3E recommended that I contact you about opportunities in the occupational health department."

Then go on to say something positive about the facility or the company as appropriate. For example, you might say, "I have always heard wonderful things about County General and would be proud to call myself a CG employee."

If you are applying for a position in sales, marketing, or training for a particular product, you might say something like, "Data Scan monitors are a superior product, and I'd love to help you spread the word."

If applying to work in a particular department or service, you might say, "Psychiatric services at County General have an outstanding reputation. I'd love to contribute to that reputation."

The Body

The second paragraph should briefly summarize your qualifications and mention what unique skills and attributes you would bring to the position. This is your chance to let the reader know why you are well suited to the position, and why you are interested in it. This is also your opportunity to add relevant information that may not be on your résumé or that needs to be elaborated on, such as relevant classes attended, related volunteer work, etc. Keep your comments brief and to the point.

The Close

End the letter on an upbeat note. Say something like, "I look forward to hearing from you so we can discuss our mutual interests further." You can include a statement about the best time and place to reach you if appropriate, such as, "Please feel free to contact me on my cell phone at 808-555-6333. Should you reach my voice mail, please leave your message and contact number, and I'll surely return your call."

End the letter with "Sincerely" (be sure to spell it correctly!) or "Yours Truly." Type your name several lines down, and sign the cover letter above your typed name.

Additional Tips

1. Print your cover letter on the same stationary as your résumé. If you have your résumé printed at a print shop, purchase extra sheets of matching paper to have available for cover letters. Be sure to create a heading at the top of the page that includes you name and address.

2. Your cover letter must always be word-processed and never handwritten. Keep it to one page.

3. Use an assertive, confident tone throughout. Rather than saying, "I hope you will find my experience appropriate," say something like, "I am confident that my experience and personality will make me an asset to the department."

5. As with your résumé, the paper and print quality must be top-notch, and the document must be free of errors. Don't rely on the grammar and spell check feature on your computer. Have someone else look it over before sending.

6. Use a conversational tone. Don't use stilted language, such as, "Enclosed herewith please find my résumé." That is the language of legal documents, and I don't know anyone other than attorneys who can decipher it. Write as you speak. Make the tone upbeat and lively. (See examples.)

7. Never use generic cover letters that you have mass-produced. These are insulting to the reader (they are detected immediately) and will likely cause your paperwork to be tossed. You've got to personalize the cover letter when possible, and always customize it to the particular position.

A nurse actively seeking work showed me the worst example of a generic cover letter I ever saw. She had a pack of preprinted form letters addressed, "To whom it may concern," with varying dates, such as, "Spring 2005," "Fall 2005," and so on. This nurse had four versions with identical

Long before computers were the norm, many others and I had to plunk out a cover letter and résumé on an old fashioned typewriter. During one particular job search, I was sending out résumés and cover letters and never getting any response. I thought that was strange since I had never had difficulty finding a job in the past. I was discussing this with a friend, and she asked to see my résumé, so I showed it to her along with a copy of a standard cover letter I was sending out. She read it through and noted that I misspelled the word "Sincerely" in my closing (I left out the second 'e'). Spelling was never one of my strong points, and I foolishly did not have someone else look the letters over. Employers were probably thinking, "How sincere can she be if she can't even spell the word right?"

content but each for a different season. She had been using this "cover letter" to enclose with her résumé when responding to classified ads or randomly sending them to local hospitals. She wondered why she wasn't getting any responses. A résumé writing service had done these for the nurse so she would have a volume of cover letters for the entire year! I guess they thought her job search would take a long time. Ironically, her search *was* taking a long time, no doubt, because of the generic letter.

Questions About Cover Letters

Q: *Classified ads often say they will only consider résumés that include salary history. How do I list that?*

A: Don't ever list your exact salary history on your résumé or in a cover letter. Instead, write something in your cover letter like, "Over the last 10 years I have been making a progressively increasing salary. I am currently earning in the mid 50s with benefits." This indicates that your total compensation package is worth more than $50,000 because your benefits have a dollar value, too. Remember: Don't mention salary AT ALL unless an ad specifically requests it.

Q: *What if an ad says that I should include my salary requirements? How do I respond to that?*

A: First, understand that there is a difference between "salary history" and "salary requirements." Employers ask these questions in an effort to determine if salary will be a stumbling block in the hiring process. Since you know very little about the position specifics at this point in time, the best way to respond to this question in writing or on the phone, if asked, is to say something like, "At this point, my salary requirements are negotiable. I need to know more about the position scope and responsibilities. I'm confident that salary won't be an obstacle." You are simply giving the employer some assurance that you are a reasonable person and need more information.

Note: The issue of salary — when to bring it up, what to say when asked about it, and why you shouldn't bring it up at this phase of the job search, will be discussed at length in chapters 7 and 8.

Q: *I've been out of the work force for a while. How do I account for that on my résumé or cover letter? Should I even mention it?*

A: You should address a current, significant absence from the workforce in your cover letter, *not* on your résumé. You can address this in the second paragraph of the letter by saying something like, "Although I have been on a recent hiatus from healthcare, I have kept current with issues and practice through contacts, associations, and continuing education."

Note: If you haven't taken steps to get up-to-date, you'll learn how to do that in Chapter 8. It is not necessary to address past lapses in employment in a cover letter. This may come up on an interview, and you can address it then. (See Chapter 7.)

Sending Out Your Résumé or CV

Unless specifically requested to fax or e-mail, it is preferable in most cases to mail your résumé or CV and cover letter via the U.S. Postal Service (USPS). This is because a well-crafted and printed hard copy document can make a more powerful first impression than an online version, and first impressions do matter. To underscore this point, think of reading a book online versus having the book in your hands. The content is the same, but the actual book has weight to it, a certain feel and look, a unique character. Online, everything looks the same. Don't underestimate the power of tactile and visual senses in making a favorable first impression.

Another reason to send a hard copy résumé is that you are more in control of what the receiver will get than you are with faxes and e-mails. For example, when documents are faxed, they often come out on the receiving end crooked, blurred, or with vital information cut off. Documents sometimes get jammed on the other end and, if sending to a large company or office with a high volume of incoming faxes, the fax may not even make it to the intended recipient. And unfortunately, you often have no way to verify that the paperwork was received intact, or that it got to the right person.

My experience has been that the U.S. Postal Service is more reliable than many fax machines.

While it is perfectly acceptable to fold a hard copy of the résumé and cover letter in thirds and mail them in a matching business size envelope, another approach would be to mail your unfolded résumé and cover letter in a white 9" X 12" envelope. Why? For starters, your submission will stand out from the others. An unfolded document makes a more professional presentation. Additionally, it will not automatically fold up on the recipient's desk thereby making it easier to read and handle. An unfolded document is also easier to file, photocopy, and electronically scan. And since an unfolded document is preferable for electronic scanning as mentioned on page 135, yours will be ready for that, too.

Note: Be sure to use the extra postage required for this size envelope. If your résumé is returned to you 10 days later with "Postage due" or if it is delivered "Postage due" to the recipient, it's all over for you. Also, type up a peel-off label for the address you are sending it to and for your return address. If using a business size envelope, you can type the address directly on the envelope.

Enclose your business card (see Chapter 10) if you have one. If sending a folded document, you can simply enclose the business card in the center. If sending unfolded documents, paper clip the card to the cover letter, or it may get lost in the envelope.

There are times when you will want or need to fax or e-mail your résumé to someone. For example, you may be responding to a classified ad that only provides a fax number for contact — no address, no employer's name, no phone number or e-mail address. In that case, you have no choice but to fax your résumé. Also, if you're working with a recruiter or prospective employer who wants to see your résumé quickly, it's OK to fax or e-mail it to them if they request you do so. But it's still a good idea to follow that up with a hard copy.

When requested to e-mail your résumé, unless specified, always ask, "Should I send my résumé as an attachment or in the body of the e-mail?" It is never a good idea to send an attachment without permission or unless requested to do so. If someone wants it as an attachment, you can simply attach your Word or Word Perfect document from your computer file. If they want it in the body of the e-mail, some reformatting will be required. E-mailing your résumé can be tricky because some formatting characteristics can be lost or can shift in transmission, especially if the recipient has a different operating system than you do. Again, include a cover letter as a separate attachment or in the body of the e-mail.

Do not include a photograph of yourself when applying for a job. Some people think this will give them a competitive edge. However, this is considered inappropriate since one could suggest that prejudicial screening was done based on someone's looks, race, ethnicity, or age.

Reminder: Whether mailing, faxing, or e-mailing your résumé or CV in response to a job opening, always include a cover letter printed on the same stationary as the résumé, except in the exclusions listed above. Remember: Your cover letter serves as your introduction and states your specific interest.

Posting Your Résumé on the Internet

In this electronic age we live in, it is common for job seekers to post their résumés online in the hopes that prospective employers or professional recruiters will find them and want to contact them. Many employers and recruiters search online résumé databanks to find job candidates. And since it is advisable to use every source available to you in a job search campaign, the Internet can give your search an extra reach.

Numerous websites facilitate job searching and career management and allow you to post your résumé at no cost. While many career sites are general in nature, some are industry specific, such as those for nursing, healthcare technology, the pharmaceutical industry, etc. Some professional association web sites offer this feature to their members. Each site has it's own procedure to follow for posting and submitting information. There is generally a form to fill out to create your online résumé.

Most forms will request that you complete a keyword section. Since a prospective employer cannot possibly read all of the online résumés posted on any given site, they will search the database for keywords to help them find people with certain qualifications, credentials, skills, and attributes they are looking for. Therefore, you must carefully choose keywords that reflect your background, especially as they relate to a particular industry or specialty you are targeting. The right keywords can determine if your résumé is identified for further scrutiny or gets lost in cyberspace.

When choosing keywords, think of words or phrases that a prospective employer might search for. Read classified ads, both print and online, and notice the words and terms that are commonly listed in the type of position you are seeking.

While industry jargon and undefined abbreviations would not normally be used in a paper résumé, they are both necessary and useful in an online résumé where keyword searches are conducted. Be sure to use only common and universally recognized abbreviations, such as ACLS, NICU, OSHA, and PACU.

Here are some examples:

- Credential keywords might include: RN, BSN, CPR certified, ACLS, CPHQ (Certified Professional in Healthcare Quality), IV certified, and MS Healthcare Management.

- Since there are so many different credential acronyms for nurse practitioners (PNP, APRN, CFNP), include the acronym but also use the key phrase "nurse practitioner." You don't want to be overlooked just because the employer didn't search for your particular credential acronym.

- Experience keywords might include: critical care, pediatrics, chemotherapy administration, oncology, trauma, outside sales, telephone triage, poison control, case management, quality improvement, phlebotomy, substance abuse, administration, management, education, clinical research, ventilator management, community outreach, managed care, and regulatory compliance.

- Skill keywords might include: public speaking, teaching, bilingual/Spanish, counseling, project management, verbal/written communication skills, training, program development, computer skills, and interpersonal skills.

- Keywords for other important traits might include: detail-oriented, self-starter, high-energy, team player, creative, independent, willing to travel, willing to relocate, dynamic, flexible, and highly motivated.

- Use short and common phraseology, like "home infusion therapy" rather than "intravenous therapy in a patient's home."

Some additional tips and information about posting your résumé online:

- Examine the online form, see what information and format is required, and then prepare your responses in a Word or Word Perfect document and save it. Then you can cut and paste it into the online form. Creating a word document first allows you to spell-check the content (online forms don't allow you to do that). You'll also have a record of the content you sent and will be able to use that content again for another form rather than having to recreate the content each time you submit an online résumé.

- Some job sites allow you to conceal your identity so that you will not be recognized by your employer (or others) if they happen to search the database you are listed on. In this case, you would be indirectly contacted by interested parties, can see who the prospective employer or recruiter is, and then opt to respond or not to that inquiry. Some sites also allow you to list search exclusions so that if your employer were searching for a particular type of candidate, your résumé would not come up when searched by that employer. (Users of the database generally have to register and log on before searching and so would be known to the system.)

- Since some employers and recruiters will search only for new résumé postings, sometimes it can be beneficial to remove your résumé from a particular database and then resubmit it if it has been online for awhile. Be sure to keep the information, including the contact information, current at all times.

Adapting Your Résumé for Scanning

Occasionally a prospective employer will advertise for, or request, a "scannable" résumé; that is, one that is adapted for electronic scanning. This process involves placing the résumé into a scanning machine, which replicates the document for storage on a computer disc. The paper document can then be discarded, thus reducing the paper volume in the office.

Usually, an employer will specify what is needed for the document to be scannable. The general rule of thumb is: no bolding of characters, no bullets, no folds in the document, 12-point type size, white paper, and black ink. Any format of résumé or CV can be adapted to become scannable. You don't need to change the layout or content of your résumé in any way. You simply need to eliminate the undesirable features, adjust the paper color and type size if necessary, and send the document unfolded. It is ONLY necessary to adapt your document for scanning if you have been specifically requested to do so.

Portfolios

A portfolio is another valuable professional tool. It is not a single document like the résumé or CV. Rather, it is a compilation of information and supporting documentation that chronicles your professional history and demonstrates your ongoing professional development.

A professional portfolio serves several purposes:

- It is a good way to keep important documents and records in one convenient and organized place.

- It maps the course of a nurse's professional life.

- It supports and enhances a résumé or CV.

- It can be used to market special skills and experiences (writing, teaching, management).

- It serves as a tool for nurses to assess their practice and skills and plan for the future.

- It is a way of documenting what you do.

While it is not necessary to bring a portfolio to a typical job interview unless asked, a portfolio may be requested for consideration of admission to graduate school and when applying for certain positions and promotions. In these cases, you would be advised what to include in your portfolio.

Some organizations use portfolios for annual evaluations and for clinical ladder programs. Some states are considering requiring nurses to keep a portfolio as a record of clinical competency and professional development for license renewal. Even if you aren't required to produce a portfolio for any of the above reasons, it is still something every nurse should consider developing. At the very least, a portfolio is a good way to keep professional documents, records, and information organized and to keep track of career specifics that go beyond your résumé or CV.

Start Simple When Putting Your Portfolio Together

Gather all your appropriate paperwork. Use a three-ring binder with plastic insert pages or a pocket folder for the material you want to include. Categorize your information, and arrange it according to some of the topics that follow. An accordion folder can help you initially get your paperwork in order and serve to hold excess or back-up documentation, such as individual CE certificates, since you would only put a listing of CE courses, not all the certificates, in a presentation portfolio. A portfolio should be arranged so that it could be presented to another professional for review if necessary.

The content of your portfolio may vary depending on the specific use. However, it is wise to accumulate all of the information below since you never know how you may want or need to use it in the future.

Formal Education: Compile diplomas, courses taken, and transcripts. Consider including a summary or abstract of any research projects done, including a thesis or dissertation. Include special papers and presentations.

Professional Credentials: Make copies of your professional licenses and certifications, including skills certifications (CPR, IV) and specialty certifications. This is an easy way to keep track of renewal dates and keep everything together in one convenient spot.

Continuing Education (CE): Keep an annual summary of all courses taken, not just clinical courses. Include programs provided by your employer as well as online and live classes you have taken. Be sure to include non-credit courses taken, certificate programs, etc. Keep course certificates in your accordion folder for reference and for presentation if requested.

Evaluations: Keep copies of annual reviews and performance appraisals. You are entitled to them, and should make it your business to get them. And while you want to keep all of them for your personal records, include only favorable reviews in a portfolio you are presenting for employment, promotion, etc. unless specifically asked to do otherwise. Also include complimentary letters received from patients or clients.

References: Keep letters of reference and your supervisor's contact information. (See section on "References" below.)

Publications: Include a listing of all published articles whether online or in print. List related work, such as book chapters written, etc.

Presentations: Document formal presentations you have given at conferences, meetings, and symposiums as well as grand rounds, community education, and in-services.

Samples of your work: Keep examples of teaching tools, flow sheets, forms, and any other education, marketing, or administrative tools and documents you have designed, developed, or written. Also include a sampling of items that demonstrate your writing style, such as articles, white papers, reports, or proposals.

Professional affiliations: List memberships, offices and positions held, committee work, and special projects and programs worked on.

Awards: Include awards and special recognition from employers, professional associations, community groups, and other agencies. This includes service awards and perfect attendance awards.

Other professional activities: Keep a record of interdisciplinary committees you have sat on and community projects you participated in, including public screening programs and health fairs. Document teaching and training activities including precepting new hires and working with students. Don't forget patient and family teaching activities. (See Skills Inventory on page 115.)

Work schedule: Keep track of how many hours you've worked in a particular job, as this can become an issue with relicensing in some states now and in the future. For example, some states require that you work a certain number of clinical hours or "hours in nursing" to be eligible for licensure renewal. You may also want to keep track of how many hours you engage in specialized activities, such as diabetic education or wound care, since that information may be required if you decide to pursue certification in these and other specialties.

Volunteer activities: List all volunteer activities, hours of service, and special projects.

Accomplishments: Keep a special section on important projects and programs that you initiated, administrated, managed, or were a key player in. Include media events, starting up new departments, and major reorganization projects, which you might have been involved in.

Annual professional goals: Every nurse should set professional goals each year and then evaluate those goals annually. Goals might be related to education, experience, skills development, professional association involvement, certification, and clinical competencies. We'll discuss goal-setting more in Chapter 10.

Because nurses are notorious for underestimating their own skills and taking their accomplishments for granted, many experts recommend designing a worksheet that you can complete annually for your own records. The worksheet could include various categories to help you reflect on your experiences. For example, you might have a section on "management experience" where you would list any charge or supervisory experience you had, as well as budgeting, scheduling, and personnel responsibilities. This type of review could also assist you in identifying transferable skills, something nurses are not generally very good at. This worksheet can also help when updating your résumé.

References

Personal and professional references have become more important than ever in a job search. Most employers wish to take every possible precaution to ensure that the person they are about to offer a job to is not only competent and reliable, but also of good moral character. Therefore, whom you choose to provide as a reference is important. But even more important is how you treat your references since this can make all the difference in the type of recommendation you get from them.

Prospective employers may request personal and/or professional references. If they don't specify, ask, because there is a difference between the two. Professional references include people you have worked with and for, who can attest to your level of experience; work habits; and how you get along with peers, subordinates, and superiors. Think of someone you've had a good working relationship with. Obviously, that person should be fairly familiar with your work. Many employers prefer to speak to an immediate supervisor, if possible.

Personal references, on the other hand, are people who have known you outside of work through your community, neighborhood, religious groups, professional associations, clubs, etc. These people can vouch for your character, personality, habits, etc. The more power and prestige the reference has, the more credible the recommendation will be. For example, a religious leader, community leader, educator, or prominent person in healthcare or business is viewed favorably. You may be asked to provide two to three references in each category.

Once you've identified the people you'd like to use, contact them and let them know you are launching a job search. Request their permission to list them as a reference and ask if they would give you a favorable reference if contacted by a prospective employer. This is important for several reasons. First, it is the courteous and considerate thing to do. Secondly, some people may not be comfortable providing a reference for you for a variety of reasons, in which case they will likely politely decline. It's better to know that up front than risk having a reference say less than favorable things about you to a prospective employer.

When it comes time to actually provide the reference's name to a prospective employer, contact the reference and let him or her know what position(s) you're applying for. Discuss the important characteristics of the job so they can highlight these things if they receive a call. Remind your references of your more significant accomplishments. Remind professional references of your title and duties while working for or with them. You should also send your references a copy of your updated résumé. Not only is this a great way to network (e.g. it keeps you fresh in their mind — they may know someone looking to hire someone with your background), but it will also remind your references of your dates of employment, job titles, projects, duties, etc. In other words, do everything you can to assist your references in giving you a top-notch recommendation! No one can remember everything about every person that ever worked for them or about everyone who asks them for a reference.

Follow-up is a must with references and yet is so often neglected by the job seeker. Keep in periodic touch with your references to let them know what's happening. If you know they were contacted for a particular job, let them know the outcome either way. Definitely let them know when you accept a position. Take time to formally thank them afterwards with a note or letter for agreeing to be a reference even if they were never called. In other words, let your references know that you appreciate them and their willingness to help out. It is also a good idea to stay in touch with your references even when you are not looking for a job.

Letters of Reference

Mobility characterizes today's workplace, especially in the nursing community. It is not uncommon for nurses to change jobs every few years or so. So when you are asked for professional references from a particular job, it is entirely possible that the person you reported to, as well as other superiors, is no longer there. You may be able to track them down through networking but that is not always possible or practical. That's why it's a good idea to get a letter of reference from your immediate supervisor when you leave a job. This way, you'll have something to show a prospective employer in the event you or they cannot connect with your work references.

As a general rule, letters of reference are not required in a job search process except in the above situation. Therefore, it is not necessary or recommended to send out unsolicited letters of reference when applying for a job. Some prospective employers do not put much stock in them.

Good references are a valuable resource. Don't take them for granted. I have often been contacted over the years to be a personal or professional reference for former employees, colleagues, and friends. I am embarrassed when called about someone I know when I didn't even know they were looking for a job! I'm sure the caller can hear my hesitation. Likewise, I appreciate it when someone who has asked me to be a reference provides me with all of the necessary information about themselves and the position(s) they are applying for. It makes my life so much easier, and they are inclined to get a better, more accurate recommendation because I am more prepared. I have also been contacted by employers to provide a reference for people about whom I have very few good things to say. If these people had at least contacted me beforehand, I would have been better prepared to discuss their strengths and weaknesses or could have politely declined to act as a reference for them. Getting caught off guard is never a good thing.

Abbreviated CV Sample

Manuel Hernandez, RN, PhD
200 Center Street
Philadelphia, PA 00070
Phone: 500-555-0396 Fax: 500-555-3013
mhernandez@net.net

EDUCATION

PhD in Nursing, Regional University, Philadelphia, PA   1996
Dissertation: New Graduate Nurse Attrition: Causes and Cures

MSN, Regional University, Philadelphia, PA   1989
Major: Adult Health and Illness   Functional Minor: Education
Thesis: Dietary Impact of Type II Diabetes Occurrence in Hispanic Population of
   Philadelphia's 3rd Ward

BSN with High Honors, Harbor University, Baltimore, MD   1985

ACADEMIC TEACHING EXPERIENCE

Professor of Nursing, County College   2004-present
   Fundamentals of nursing, senior leadership practicum, community health
Acting Chairperson, Department of Nursing, Mid-State College   Spring 2003
Assistant Professor of Nursing, Mid-State College   1996-2004
   Course and curriculum development in new BSN program
Instructor — College of Nursing, Downstate University   1992-1996
   Lecture and clinical supervision related to "Nursing Process in Secondary Care"

Teaching/research interests: Shared governance, medical ethics, nursing leadership

PROFESSIONAL EXPERIENCE

Maryland County Hospital   Medical/Surgical Nursing   1989-1994
Carter Memorial Hospital   Medical/Surgical Nursing   1985-1989
Mid-State Army Hospital   U.S. Army Reserves, CCU, MICU   1985-1989

SELECTED PUBLICATIONS

Hernandez, C. & Waters, J. (2007). Second Career Nursing Students; Challenges and
   Opportunities. *American Nurse Today,* 4(8), 60-64.
Hernandez, C. (2006). Shared Governance in Practice. *Nurse Leader,* 10(4), 24-28.
Hernandez, C. (2005). An Ethical Discussion about End of Life Care. *American Journal of
   Nursing,* 12(3), 8-16.

SELECTED PRESENTATIONS

"Using Leadership to Enhance Your Clinical Practice," Emergency Nurses Association
   Leadership Conference, February 2007, Boston, MA
"How to Apply for the Magnet Award," New Jersey Nursing Convention, March, 2007,
   Atlantic City, NJ

Sample Cover Letter
SHEILA WATSON, RN
45 Lane Avenue
Smithville, New Jersey 00090
908-555-2222 Cell 908-333-5555
swatson@net.net

November 8, 20___

Harold Meyers, RN
Nurse Recruiter
Cantor Medical Center
55 Main Street
Wall, IL 00875

Dear Mr. Meyers,

I am enthusiastically applying for the position of Staff Nurse, Medical-Surgical Unit, as advertised in the *Gazette* on November 7. I've met many nurses who work at Cantor Medical, and they all speak very highly of the facility and its management team. I would be proud to call myself a Cantor Nurse.

I am an RN with 2 years of medical/surgical experience currently working in a small community hospital. Working at Cantor, a teaching hospital, would expand my horizons and my opportunities. My good work ethic, passion for nursing, and readiness to take my career to the next level would make me an asset to the nursing team. Additionally, I am always working on professional development and am planning to enter a BSN program in the future.

I look forward to meeting with you so that we can discuss our mutual interests further. You may contact me by phone or e-mail as I will be checking both for messages regularly. Thank you in advance!

Sincerely,

Sheila Watson, RN

Sheila Watson, RN

Sample New Graduate Cover Letter
Carl Fuller, RN
45 Lane Avenue
Smithville, New Jersey 00090
908-555-2222
carfull@net.net

November 8, 20___

Harold Meyers, RN
Nurse Recruiter
Cantor Medical Center
55 Main Street
Wall, IL 00875

Dear Mr. Meyers,

I am a new graduate nurse with his sites set on working at Cantor Medical Center. I did a pediatric rotation there while attending County College School of Nursing and was very impressed with everyone I met. It was easy to see why Cantor has a reputation for providing excellent nursing care. I can't think of a better place to start my nursing career.

While working as an Emergency Medical Technician (EMT) on a volunteer ambulance service, I developed a keen interest in emergency room nursing and am most interested in opportunities in that department. However, I am open to other opportunities at CMC. I saw on your web site that you offer a special new graduate orientation program along with specialty internships. That was particularly appealing to me. My high energy, attention to detail, and readiness to roll up my sleeves and work hard would be an asset to your organization.

I would relish the opportunity to discuss with you how I can best contribute to Cantor's great reputation as well as what Cantor Medical Center has to offer a new graduate nurse like me. Thank you for your consideration. I eagerly await your reply.

Yours truly,

Carl Fuller, RN

Carl Fuller, RN

Interviewing

There was a time in nursing when you could pretty much just show up at a hospital, state that you were a nurse, and get hired almost on the spot. I always joke that the only question we were asked on a job interview in the old days was, "When can you start?" Of course those days are long gone, and nurses need to learn the fine art of self-marketing.

The thought of going on a job interview makes most people turn pale, get diaphoretic, and develop cold and clammy skin. The spotlight is on you during an interview, and most of us have difficulty talking about ourselves in a positive way. Nurses, generally, are not comfortable "selling" themselves, and that is exactly what you are doing on an interview: pointing out the benefits to the buyer, overcoming objections, and closing the sale. That's sales lingo, but it's exactly what you have to do.

The good news is that although individual interviewer style and format may vary, you can significantly improve your ability to interview well by learning and practicing the art and science of competitive interviewing. An interview is not simply a random question and answer session between two strangers. There is much more technique involved than most nurses realize. Once you understand the elements of an effective interview, learn to answer commonly asked questions, and get a little practice, you'll be able to interview with the best of them.

An interview is a time-honored ritual used for both parties to obtain further information. Each party has an objective and an ideal outcome. Your objective is twofold: to present yourself and your background in the best possible light and to get more information about the job, the company, and of course to ultimately get a job offer. You are evaluating a particular position and employer and trying to determine if the position offers the opportunities, circumstances, challenges, and compensation that you want and need. The interviewer's objective is to determine if you can do this job and do it well, if you are interested and excited about it, if there are any potential problems in your background, and to see if you will fit in and contribute to the employer's success. An interview is very much a two way street.

It is important to understand that a job interview is a formal workplace situation and should be treated as such. It is not a casual social call. Therefore, you should dress your best, be on your best behavior at all times, conduct yourself professionally at every stage of the process, be well prepared, and keep your guard up at all times. More on all that in a moment.

There are several different types of interviews, which we'll discuss a little later in the next chapter. For the moment, let's focus on the traditional hiring interview, where you meet face to face with the person or persons for whom you would be directly working. Note: The preparation advice below applies to almost all interview situations.

Preparation

It is not always the best-qualified candidate but often the best-prepared candidate that lands a job. Likewise, if there are several equally qualified candidates for a job, it is likely the one that is best prepared for the interview that will be chosen. Preparation for a job interview is key to your success. Here's what you need to do.

Ask the Right Questions

When you are contacted to set up an interview, ask, "Who will be interviewing me?" Be sure to get the names and titles of everyone who will be

"Sometimes employers' schedules change without notice; the initial plan is to interview with HR and the manager separately but [you] might end up interviewing with both at the same time. The interviewee should be prepared and flexible if this occurs and not get freaked out. The interviewee's reaction to this unplanned situation will be observed. Remember the saying: it is not what happens to you so much as how you react to the situation!"

— Agnes, Nurse Recruiter

interviewing you. You'll want to determine if this is a screening interview with a nurse recruiter or someone in Human Resources or if this is a hiring interview with a direct supervisor or manager. In some cases, more than one person will be interviewing you either separately or as a group. It is important to know this going in so you won't be surprised. Don't be afraid to ask these questions. They are expected and they show you are intelligent and savvy about the interview process.

Do Your Homework

Before any interview, research the position, the specialty if applicable, and the employer (facility, company, agency). Research the employer by asking for some corporate literature to be sent to you, such as an annual report or marketing material. You can also offer to stop by and pick it up at an earlier date. If you do this, be sure to dress professionally and be courteous and professional to everyone you meet in the process. Just running in to pick something up doesn't mean that it's OK to show up in shorts or a sweat suit.

While you're at it, see if you can get a copy of the job description of the position for which you're applying. Also ask that any additional required paperwork, such as a job application, be sent beforehand if possible. This way you can fill it out at your leisure and have one less thing to do on the big day.

Visit the employer's website. Read their mission statement, press releases, etc. Visit the prospective employee (Work for Us) page, etc.

Just as you might do an Internet search to see what turns up about a prospective employer and the interviewer, it is common for prospective employers to do an Internet search for your name to see what comes up. I recently heard from two recruiters who did an Internet search on two different job candidates and came up with information about prior arrests. If the information is out there, you need to know about it and be prepared to address it.

Also, everything you write in a chat room, blog, your own home page on a networking site, etc. is searchable and can influence a prospective employer. Some employers will go to specific popular sites and search for any posts by you. Search for your own name on the Internet and on various sites you contribute to, to see what comes up. Post on the Internet responsibly or don't use your real name when doing so. Always consider how what you write might affect you at a later time.

Observe what, if anything, the website says about the nursing staff and about their employees, benefits, philosophy, etc. Note their accreditation status if applicable, the size of the facility or agency, how old the organization is, and so on.

Do an Internet search for additional information about the employer and the person who will be interviewing you. Look for news stories and other related links and information. You never know what you'll turn up. Then, during the interview, find subtle ways to mention some things you learned online. The interviewer will be impressed that you made the effort to do your homework. At the very least, you will be armed with more knowledge about the prospective employer and the interviewer(s).

Activate your network (ask around) to find anyone who now works for or has worked for the organization that you will be interviewing with. Ask them about the company and the department. Also, seek out information about the person you would be working directly for and the person who would be hiring you, if different. Try to find out about their management style, their reputation, and their particular likes and dislikes in the workplace. Even if you want to keep your job search confidential, you can confide in a few close friends or family members and ask them to keep your name out of it when making inquiries.

To learn more about the specialty in general as well as the particular position you're applying for, do some informational interviewing with others in a similar position in a similar work setting. (Refer to Chapter 3.)

Scout Out the Location

Be sure you know the exact location of the interview and how to get there. Make a dry run beforehand, if necessary, during the same time of day as your interview appointment.

I was recently in a downtown area store when a young woman came running in frantically saying she had an interview at 23 Front Street (the street we were on) and none of the buildings had the number 23 on them. No one in the store could help her, no one had heard of the company she was looking for, and she did not bring the phone number with her. She was already late and totally panic struck. I don't know the outcome, but it couldn't have been good.

Prepare Yourself

Take inventory of your strengths and assets. Write them down on an index card (or two). This way you can review them just before the interview (take them with you) so they'll be fresh in your mind. Review your résumé and background especially as it relates to this position. Be prepared to discuss similar types of work you have done, especially when applying for a position in a new specialty or work setting.

Rehearse answers to commonly asked and anticipated questions until you feel comfortable and confident. Consider role-playing the interview with a friend or family member or rehearsing your responses aloud in front of a mirror so as to also observe your facial expression and body language. Some nurses have gone on interviews for positions that they're not too interested in, just to get the interview practice before the real thing comes along.

Start getting yourself pumped up and positive before, and the day of, the interview. Listen to motivational tapes, read motivational articles and books, and use positive self-talk. Use visualization to imagine your desired outcome. Example: Picture yourself looking and feeling confident and sharp, answering each anticipated question with ease, getting a great job offer, and generally going through the interview process with panache. Do all this for several days before if possible. Listen to something upbeat as you drive to the interview, such as a favorite tape or the theme song from the movie *Rocky*. These things will help you to stay positive and focused; they really work!

What to Bring

Since you want to be well prepared for anything that might come up, bring extra copies of your résumé, business cards, and a small notebook if you wish to jot down notes and information and to have prepared questions written down. The extra résumés come in handy if the interviewer can't find the one that you previously sent (It happens!), or if you meet other key people while there who ask if you have an extra copy. All of this shines a positive light on you and shows that you are organized, that you plan ahead, and are well prepared. You can carry all of this in a professional folder.

Upon Arrival

Allow yourself more than enough time to get there to account for any potential problems, such as traffic delays, getting lost, finding parking, etc. (Make sure you have enough gas in the car and bring along the phone num-

• •

Force yourself to smile even before the interview so your brain starts to become more positive. Of course, you don't want to have a nervous smile plastered on your face, but try to smile naturally. Stand tall with shoulders back and head upright. You don't have to actually be confident to look and act confident. Take a few deep breaths and go for it!

• •

ber of the person who will be interviewing you just in case!) You should arrive in enough time to be able to go into the restroom and check your appearance, have a few moments to compose yourself, and otherwise get yourself together. Check your hair and makeup or tie, dry your hands if your palms are sweaty, review your notes and your strengths and assets if necessary, and do one final round of positive self-talk or affirmations, such as, "I am an experienced, competent, and capable person."

If you're wearing an outer coat, take it off and carry it over your left arm so your right hand is free to shake hands. Unless you have been advised to come in early to fill out an application, wait until 10 or 15 minutes before your appointment time to announce your arrival to the receptionist. If you arrive very early, wait quietly in an inconspicuous place such as your car or an outside bench, allowing enough time to get yourself together and focused.

When you arrive, understand that you are being evaluated every step of the way, so be on your best behavior and be courteous to everyone you meet, including the parking lot attendant, receptionist, security guard, etc. People talk to other people. It's not uncommon for a manager to ask a receptionist, "What did you think of that candidate?" because how a person acts with ancillary staff can offer good insight to that person's true personality and character.

Elements of a Successful Interview

The Introduction

The first few seconds of any interview are critical. First impressions are made in as little as three seconds, and once they are in place, they are lasting and difficult to shake. Upon meeting the person who will be interviewing you, stand up (if seated), make immediate eye contact, smile naturally, and shake hands firmly. (See Chapter 10.) This brief three step process (handshake, eye contact, smile) can make or break an interview — it's that important. Extend your hand to shake even if the interviewer doesn't.

It is said that prospective employers make a preliminary decision within the first two minutes of meeting you as to whether or not they will likely hire you. That doesn't mean that the interviewer has decided whether or not they like you, but they do get a preliminary sense about who you are and whether or not you are someone who is confident, competent, credible, and personable. We'll discuss overall appearance and what to wear in Chapter 8.

Once the introduction is made, the interviewer may ask if you had any trouble finding the place. Respond by saying something benign like, "None at all, thank you. The directions were great." Use this response regardless of the reality, even if the directions were terrible, or you got horribly lost. You don't want to offer any negatives into the interview process, especially not right in the beginning. And at this point, it really doesn't matter. The question is more of a polite opener rather than a query requiring a factual answer.

The Warm-Up

If the interviewer has come to walk you to the interview room, necessitating a brief walk together, you want to engage in small talk with him or her during this time. Small talk is that light, superficial banter we engage in when we meet people for the first time or see someone we know. While some people view small talk as a meaningless time waster, in reality it serves a very important social function and should not be ignored or downplayed. It allows people an opportunity to warm up to each other before getting into more serious conversation. It even allows both parties to get accustomed to the sound of the other's voice through light conversation before discussing more serious matters.

Take an active role in this, without chattering nonstop, rather than standing silently by and letting the interviewer do all the talking. You do want to let the interviewer set the tone for the conversation, but you don't want to be too passive, either. Here are some things you might say if the opportunity arises, "It's a lovely day out. I enjoyed the ride here," or, "This is a beautiful building. When was it built?" Keep it simple and light.

The Opener

Once seated in the location where the interview will take place (allow the interviewer to indicate where you should sit), it's time to get down to the business of getting to know one another better and finding out if the job is right for you, and if you are the right candidate for the job. And while every interviewer has his or her own style and format, a typical first question is something such as, "Tell me about your self."

This type of open-ended question is often asked simply to get you talking so the interviewer can get a sense of who you are and what your personality is like. Keep your response to this question light and brief, about two minutes in length, describing what you're doing now and what you've done in the recent past. Restrict your comments to professional work and activities and avoid personal disclosures. If you're not currently working or haven't worked in the recent past, you can talk about your career prior to that. Keep in mind that this is just an opening overview. There will be plenty of time to get into specifics later.

• •
Be prepared with a list of questions you want to ask.
• •

While the interviewer is listening to what you have to say, she will also be observing your nonverbal communication cues (body language, eye contact, facial expressions, hand gestures, etc.) throughout the interview. Some people are so nervous during an interview that they tend to clam up, get stiff, never smile, and speak in a monotone, which is not good. So here are some tips for conveying confidence, interest, intelligence, enthusiasm, honesty, and friendliness. Sit upright, leaning slightly forward. Don't sink into the chair. Make good eye contact throughout the interview without staring. Smile freely as appropriate, but not continuously. The use of hand gestures is good as long as those movements are low and close to your body. It is not necessary to clasp your hands in your lap as if you were in a grade school classroom. It is better to be a bit animated during the interview to show that you have some life and personality. However, if you are someone who gestures nervously in a distracting way, you may have to tone it down a bit. Speak in a clear, firm voice and let your personality shine through. Remember to act confident, even if you don't feel confident.

The Needs Assessment

At a convenient time during the interview, as early as possible, you should ask the interviewer something like, "I'm interested to know what you see as an ideal candidate for this job." This is an important question for several reasons. First, it shows the interviewer that you are interested in what he or she wants and needs. Secondly, it will provide you with valuable information on how to best market yourself. You can't effectively sell yourself if you don't know what the interviewer is looking for. Otherwise, you might spend time and energy talking about your certifications and experience when what the interviewer really wants is someone who doesn't call in sick all the time because that's why they had to let the last person go. So ask the question, listen attentively to the answer, think about how you fit that "ideal," and find ways to get that message across to the interviewer.

Example: In answer to your question, the interviewer responds, "Well, we need someone with good communication skills because you will be interfacing with doctors, the public, and other department members, etc." You might respond with, "That's great, because I pride myself on being able to communicate clearly and effectively with a wide range of different types of people."

Questions, Questions, and More Questions

As previously mentioned, an interview is a two-way street. You will certainly be expected to answer a certain number of questions, but you should also ask some questions other than those already mentioned above.

Ask Questions

Be prepared with a list of questions you want to ask about the job and the company. It is perfectly acceptable to carry a small notepad on which you have listed your questions. It is also acceptable to make an occasional brief note during the course of the interview (bring your own pen). Don't get carried away with this though. You want to be making eye contact and listening, not writing throughout the interview. Asking intelligent and relevant questions shows the interviewer that you are genuinely interested in the position and have taken time to research it and formulate questions.

In the early part of the interview, while you're getting to know one another, ask clarifying questions related specifically to job duties, responsibilities, size and scope of department, reporting mechanism, etc. Here are some examples of "early" interview questions:

- What are you looking for in an ideal candidate for this job?
- Why is this position open?
- Who would I be reporting to? What is the chain of command?
- What type of orientation/training program is provided?
- Describe the department staffing.
- Would I be required to work overtime; weekends; take call?

- What type of support staff does the department have? (volunteers, unit/department secretary, aides, etc.)

Later in the interview, once you have established rapport and have had an opportunity to sell yourself, ask more pointed questions such as:

- What are the biggest challenges the department faces right now?
- What problems/issues exist in the department that would need addressing in the first two to three months? (This is appropriate if applying for a supervisory or management position.)
- Where do you see the company/department going in the next few years?
- Are there opportunities for continuing education?
- Are there any opportunities for promotion from this position?
- How would you describe your management style? (Ask this when speaking with the person you would be reporting to.)
- What are the most important traits you look for in an employee or team member? (This is different from the ideal candidate question.)
- How long have you worked here? (This can be asked of anyone who interviews you.)
- Followed by, "What do like most and least about working here?"

It is generally not appropriate to ask about salary and benefits on an initial interview. You can stop by the human resource office for some benefits information (insurance, pension, tuition reimbursement, etc.) if you wish. We will talk more about the issue of salary later.

Commonly Asked Questions

While most recruiters and some prospective employers are experienced and skilled interviewers, other employers are not experienced at interview-

Sometimes, human resources is the first stop in the interview process (completing an application, filling out background and reference check forms, etc). Every company is different in this regard. If the HR professional offers information regarding established salary and benefits, then it is perfectly appropriate to discuss and ask questions. However, all salary and benefits negotiations should be left for later in the interview process as discussed in Chapter 8.

ing and are just as nervous as you are. Many will ask questions that they, themselves, have been asked on interviews or try to come up with something that they believe will give them insight into who you are. Below are some of the most frequently asked questions by interviewers along with advice on how to best answer them.

Why do you want this job?

This is a very important question and many job candidates answer it inappropriately. Your answer must specifically relate to the job in question. That is, the interviewer is interested to know what it is about this particular job or field that you are interested in. Do not respond by relating why you want to leave your current job, or that you are simply looking for "something different." An employer wants to know that you have some concept of the job responsibilities or of the industry and that you are deliberately looking to work there rather than throwing out multiple feelers hoping someone will bite. Your interview preparation work, previously discussed in this chapter, should provide information that will allow you to formulate an appropriate response to this question.

If you're applying for a position in a specialty or work setting that is different than what you've done in the past, the interviewer will be particularly interested to know why you are interested in pursuing this type of work. So, in answer to this question you might say something like, *"I've done my own research, including speaking to several people that have been involved in this line of work. It has always sounded challenging and interesting to me, and I've decided it's something I'd like to do."*

Why do you want to work for this company/facility?

Again, the answer must relate specifically to that company or facility. Example: *"Liberty Medical has an excellent reputation in the industry, and I want to be part of this winning team."* Do not respond by saying that the location is convenient. This is not a strong enough answer. The prospective employer wants to believe that you really want to work there because you think well of the place.

What are your long and short term goals?

Keep your answer brief and general. Think in terms of what the interviewer is interested in. For example, for a long term goal, you could mention that you are planning to get back into school, if indeed you are. Otherwise, state that you would like to develop expertise in this particular field or something similar. For a short term goal, you might say that your short term goal is to land this position!

What are your best and worst points?

Your response should indicate a "best point" that is significant, such as, "My outgoing personality," or, "My ability to get along with all types of people." Your worst point should be something that could be perceived as a negative and a positive. Example: *"My worst point is probably the fact that I am too much of a perfectionist and tend to want to keep reworking projects. However, I'm working on easing up on myself in that regard."* Perfectionism can be negative, but it is really more of a positive. You have to state why it is a negative — in this case because you keep reworking things — and that you are working to improve it. Who can argue with this! Here's another "worst point" example: *"I sometimes expect too much from the people I work with. However, I'm trying to temper my expectations and appreciate that everyone works at a different pace."* Again, this is something that can be perceived as both positive and negative and ultimately will reflect positively on you. This is all part of the art and science of effective interviewing.

Why do you want to leave your current job (If currently working)?

The best way to handle this is to say something like, *"It's not that I'm looking to leave my current job, but this is something I have always wanted to do (or this is someplace I have always wanted to work), and when I heard about this opportunity, it sounded too good to pass up."* Remember, you never want to introduce any potential negatives into a job interview. Any reason you might suggest for wanting to leave your current job is a potential negative and could open a can of worms.

The only exception to this would be if you have been notified that your position or department is being eliminated, in which case you could respond with, *"I'm not looking to leave but as it turns out my department is being eliminated. Although I have always enjoyed working there, when I heard about this opportunity, I realized the timing was right for me to make my move."*

Why did you leave your last job (If you are currently not working)?

Your response will depend on the circumstances of your leaving your last job.

When answering questions, think in terms of what the interviewer is interested in hearing about. That is, keep the responses business-related for the most part. For instance, you might think that your best point is being a good parent, but this is not of particular interest to the interviewer. Remember, the employer is trying to determine if you are right for this job, and if you can do this job.

A. If you were downsized, laid off, or something similar beyond your control: *"My position/department was eliminated, and there were very few other positions to go after. While I was happy working there, I saw this occurrence as an opportunity to pursue other areas that I have been interested in for some time. That's what brings me here today."* The beauty of this response is that you have honestly stated the reason for your current unemployment while putting a positive spin on it, and you bring it right back to the job at hand. This is the art of good interviewing.

B. If you have been out of the work force for personal reasons, such as raising a family, or taking care of elderly parents or a sick relative, you can simply say, *"There were issues in my family life (or personal life) that needed my full-time attention for a while. Circumstances are different now, and I am eager to get back into the workforce."* An employee who is eager to work and not burned out is very desirable in today's marketplace.

Use a similar response to address any gaps in your employment history, even if currently employed. For example, if asked why you had a two-year gap in employment history several years ago, you could respond by saying something like, *"I took a brief hiatus from work to tend to some family matters."* You can reveal some specifics if you wish, but keep it light and superficial such as, *"I was at home raising my family during that time,"* or, *"I was caring for elderly parents."* Be sure to add, *"That is no longer an issue."*

C. If you were let go (fired) due to problems of some sort, be honest but keep it very light and put a positive spin on it. Remember this is a job interview, not a confessional!

Example #1: *"I was let go from my previous job because I had excessive absences. I had a family challenge going on, and it was difficult for me to get into work every day. In retrospect, I should have taken a leave of absence rather than trying to juggle work and other pressing matters in my life. Let me*

Be aware that some states have laws regarding disclosure of certain information by present and former healthcare employers when requested by prospective healthcare employers related to clinical practice and patient care issues. This is one reason why it is best to be honest and upfront about these situations if they exist in your employment history. If you conceal something like this and the employer finds out about it later, you will almost definitely be disqualified from the position. However, if you disclose the situation and address it adequately, the prospective employer may be willing to hire you in spite of it, depending on the situation.

Regardless of the reason you actually left, you never want to say anything negative about a former company, facility, or supervisor. It does not reflect well on you, and you will be opening a can of worms. Be professional and discreet where former employers are concerned.

assure you that the situation is now completely resolved, and I will never let that happen again."

Example #2: *I was let go after self-reporting a medication error. Fortunately, there was no harm to my patient, but the facility has a strict policy about med errors. I was trying to do too many things at once that day and should have asked for help. I learned a very hard lesson from that experience, and I assure you that it will never happen again."* Keep your facial expression neutral and steady. If you look like you're ready to bust out crying, it will scare the interviewer. Rehearse your response beforehand so you can deliver it calmly.

Example #3: If you left your last job because you just couldn't take another day there for whatever reason, it is best to respond with something such as, *"I was simply ready for a new challenge in my career and knew it would be difficult to launch a job search while working full time. I know it was a risky thing to do — quitting one job without having another one lined up — but I felt confident that I would find something suitable within a reasonable amount of time. Besides, this way I got to take a little time off to recharge my batteries so I can get started in my next position well rested."* Say this with a smile on your face.

Where do you see yourself in five years?

The best response is something like, *"I see myself doing this (whatever you are applying for) but ideally in a position of increased responsibility."* This is telling the interviewer that you have staying power, and while you would hope to be in a position of increased responsibility, as any person of average intelligence and motivation would be, you are not hell-bent on being in-charge. Never respond with, "I see myself in your job." While many people use this response and see it as clever, it is generally perceived to be rude and arrogant.

What type of salary are you looking for?

If you are asked this question at any time before or during the interview, prior to being made a job offer, respond by saying something like, *"My salary requirements are negotiable. At this time I'm more interested in knowing if the job is right for me, and if I'm the right candidate for the job."* If the interviewer pushes the issue, repeat the above and add, *"We can discuss salary if we become mutually interested in working together. Besides, I don't know enough about the position and the responsibilities yet to have a realistic expectation."*

The reality is that you can't possibly have a salary requirement before you have more in-depth information about the position you are applying for, such as if you have to do shift work or work weekends or holidays; whether there is any support staff; how big the department is in terms of number of employees, budget, volume of work, etc. All of these make a difference in how much you would reasonably expect to make. Therefore, the discussion of money is pointless at the preliminary stages of an interview.

I'm sure some of you are thinking, "But I can't afford to make less than X amount of money so why should I waste my time interviewing for the job if the salary is below what I want and need?" The answer is that you put yourself at a great disadvantage by mentioning a salary figure early on for several reasons. If you were to mention a figure that is below what the employer is offering, you can ruin your chances of getting top salary during the negotiation phase. Also, if you quote a figure well below what they traditionally pay, you may be perceived as not being at the level of experience they are looking for.

You can also hurt yourself by quoting a figure too high this early in the game and knocking yourself out of the running before you even have a chance to interview. That would be foolish on your part since, as already mentioned, there are many times that a job candidate comes in to interview for one job, and is offered a better, higher-paying job afterwards. Also, once an employer is sold on you and wants to hire you, you have some negotiation power, which you did not have early on. So even if your salary requirements are higher than what might be typically offered for this job, you are now in a better position to negotiate something that is more to your satisfaction. By contrast, you have no negotiation power early in the interview process. Once the employer is interested in you, everything changes.

In Chapter 8 we'll discuss how to respond to illegal, situational, and abstract questions.

The Home Stretch

When the interview is wrapping up (e.g., it appears that the Q&A session is over), you've gotten all of your questions answered about the position, and the interviewer seems to be winding down, there are three additional questions you should ask:

1. When might I expect to hear from you? OR When do you anticipate making a decision?

If the interviewer doesn't bring it up first, you need to ask. Typically, the interviewer, in response to your question, will give a time frame anywhere from one week to three weeks. If he or she were to say, "Gee I'm not really sure yet," you might respond, "How does two weeks sound?" The interviewer will either say, "That sounds about right," or "Give me three weeks." You should never leave an interview without a time frame for follow-up.

2. Have you interviewed anyone else yet for this position?

If the response is "No, you're the first one," move on to the next question.

If the answer is "Yes" to the above, follow it with, "Where do I stand with the competition?" Say this in a light-hearted manner with a smile on your face, not in a confrontational way.

Interviewers will likely answer in one of two ways. They'll either give you a very generalized, noncommittal response such as, "You're one of several qualified candidates I've seen so far," or they'll give you some actual comparative information that will give you a real sense of where you stand. This is a very important question to ask for two reasons. First, it shows that you are interested in the position, are assertive, and understand that you may be competing with others for this position. Secondly, if the interviewer is forthright with you, the information you obtain can be invaluable (see sidebar on page 164 of this chapter).

And last but not least...

3. Do you have any reservations about me that I can clear up before I leave today?

I'm sure some of you are thinking, "Is she nuts? I could never say something like that — I don't have the nerve. Besides, what if they say that they DO have reservations? Then what am I supposed to do?"

As scary as it might seem to ask this question, it is actually one of the best things you can do to flush out and immediately address any reservations the interviewer may actually have about you before you leave the interview. Why? Because if the interviewer does have reservations about you, even small ones, and they are not addressed at the time of the interview, those reservations will loom larger and larger as time passes. Better to nip them in the bud.

Here's an example of why it's important to ask this question as well as how to address a specific objection:

Interviewee who does not have any direct experience related to the position they're applying for: "Do you have any reservations about me that I can address before I leave today?"

Interviewer: "You seem like a really nice person, but the truth is that I was hoping to find someone with more experience in this specialty."

Interviewee: "Look at it this way: You can train me to do the job exactly the way you want it done. I'm coming to you with no bad habits and no professional baggage." Of course you would say this in a confident manner with a smile on your face.

The fact that the interviewer has some concerns about you is not a problem as long as you know what they are and can address them. As in the above example, don't expect the interviewer to think of this reason himself. You have to counter the objection and turn it into a positive. This is part of the art and science of effective interviewing. Even if the interviewer says they have no reservations (whether or not that is a true statement) the important thing is that you asked the question.

Overcoming Objections

Here are some additional responses to common objections to be used ONLY if they are brought up by the interviewer as a reservation:

No Experience

There are two approaches that you can use here, depending on the situation. If you are applying for something that will require some specialized training, such as utilization review or pharmaceutical research, and if the fact that you have no direct experience in that specialty becomes a stumbling block for the interviewer, you can take the tack previously mentioned that turns your inexperience into a positive thing:

"If you think I've got the right personality and attitude, you can always train me to do the job. You could hire someone else with experience but you can't change his or her attitude if it isn't what you're looking for."

However, in Chapter 3 we discussed all the transferable skills that nurses have, and how we tend to downplay our abilities. So don't be so quick to say that you don't have experience in something or that you've never done something before. Rather, think of some way that you've done something similar in nursing. For example, if asked if you have any experience with case management, rather than saying "no," you might say, "Although I've never had the title of case manager, I've been involved in the case manage-

● ●

It's All in How You Present Yourself

Krystyna had 15 years of clinical experience. She worked full-time in various specialties and always had part-time side jobs in different settings and specialties, such as home infusion, occupational health, and quality improvement for a physician's office.

Krystyna relates, *"While doing all that, I always kept an eye open for what was going on outside of the hospital but never had the guts to leave the 'secured place.' Being in a management position for over two years and dealing with cutting budgets, training nurses and techs to do more and more, and constantly pleasing the unsatisfied customers and miserable staff made me realize that I can do something else. I applied to an ad in* Nursing Spectrum *for medical research and was told that I had no experience. After I got off the phone, I thought about it and actually got mad. What did they mean I did not have any experience? I didn't directly do the same work but was involved in many areas of research while working in the hospital. So, out of frustration, I called them back, not thinking that would change their mind, but to tell them how much experience I actually had in that area. Much to my surprise, I was offered a job with one of the largest pharmaceutical companies in the world!"*

● ●

ment process by sitting on a discharge planning committee and having in-depth discussions with the case manager about my patients and their post-discharge needs. I've become very familiar with the case management process." In other words, think in terms of what you can do, rather than what you can't do. Revisit the section on Transferable Skills in Chapter 3 for some additional examples.

Out of Nursing for A While

If this objection comes up, the interviewer is concerned that you are not up to date with your knowledge, and he fears you may be generally out of touch with current practice. This relates to nonclinical positions, such as case management, telephone triage, or quality improvement. (Note: An absence from clinical practice has different significance and requirements when applying for a direct patient care position. We'll discuss that situation specifically in Chapter 9.)

"Let me assure you that I've kept current with issues by reading professional journals, taking continuing education courses, and staying active in my professional associations." (Hopefully you will have done some of these things in preparation for getting back into the job market.)

"Look at it this way; I'm rested, fresh, and raring to go. I'm not the least bit burned out." This can sound great to someone who is working with staff members that are burned out and apathetic.

No Degree or Not a High Enough Degree

"I understand the importance of higher education, but you have to give me credit for all of the relevant experience I do have, not to mention my passion for this work. I can always go back to school and start working on that degree, which I would be willing to do if offered this job." That can sometimes be enough to get past the degree requirement. And getting back to school would be a good thing anyway.

Sporadic Work History

Acknowledge the situation by saying something like, "Over the last ten years there were issues in my family life that periodically needed my full attention. That's all resolved now (or that's no longer an issue), and I'm ready and willing to get back on a full-time, permanent basis." You don't need to reveal any specifics. Much will depend on your demeanor and body language when you say this. If you appear nervous and avoid eye contact, it may concern the interviewer. If you seem confident and relaxed and have a smile on your face, the interviewer will hopefully accept you at your word.

Overqualified

If this objection comes up, the employer is concerned that you will not be challenged by the job, or that they cannot pay you what they think you should be making or what you've made in the past. You have to convince him or her otherwise by saying something like, "I understand how you might think that, but I see opportunity to learn and grow in this job. I'm interested and excited about it and am perfectly willing to work for the salary you're offering. Look at this way; you'll be getting good value for your money."

Remember, the fact that the employer has an objection is not the problem. You just have to convince them that whatever their concern is about you, it's not going to be a problem and may even be an asset for them. Reframe the situation for them; assure them of your value, worth, interest, and commitment to the job and move forward.

Years ago, I interviewed for a position I wanted as a department director in a community hospital. I went on an initial interview, which seemed to go very well. The person who interviewed me, a hospital vice president, told me I would receive a phone call to come back for a second interview. I left feeling rather smug, assuming that I had the job and that the second interview was likely a formality. When I received the call to arrange the second interview, I asked several key questions that I am sure helped me land the position. I first asked, "Who will be interviewing me this time?" I found out I would be interviewed by the same person as well as two other department directors that I would be working closely with. This would be done in a panel format (see Chapter 8), meaning that I would meet with everyone at the same time. This information allowed me to mentally prepare.

I also asked another critical question, "Are you bringing anyone else in for a second interview?" I needed to know if this was a formality, or if I was still competing with other candidates. The VP responded, "Yes, we are bringing back another candidate." I obviously had jumped the gun assuming I was "it." So I asked another important question, "Where do I stand with the competition?" The interviewer was frank with me and responded, "To tell you the truth, you are both very similar in personality and experience, and frankly I'm having difficulty making up my mind between the two of you." Egads! I was competing with someone so similar to myself that he couldn't even make up his mind! After my shock wore off, I sprang into mental action.

The Finale

The interviewer will signal when the interview has come to an end, usually by standing up. At this time, again shake hands, make direct eye contact, and smile. Leave on a positive note by saying something upbeat such as, "It was a pleasure to meet you. Thank you for taking the time to talk with me. I am very interested in this position, and I look forward to hearing back from you!"

People tend to remember beginnings and endings so even if the interview didn't go great, you can leave a good impression by starting and ending strong.

Additional tip: Upon leaving, ask for some corporate literature to take with you if you don't already have it, and be sure to get the interviewer(s)'s business card.

For starters, I knew I had to be extra sharp and polished on the second interview. I was being evaluated by new people and still very much in a neck-and-neck race. Had I not known this, I believe I would have been somewhat complacent and let my guard down a bit assuming I had the job in the bag. Now I did just the opposite. I knew I had to find some way to distinguish myself from this other person who I did not know anything about other than she was perceived as "very similar" to me. So I racked my brain to see what I could come up with. Here's what happened.

At the end of the second interview, after all of the traditional things were discussed, the VP asked me if I had anything else I wanted to add. This was my cue to tell them what I hoped would set me apart. I said, "I did want to mention that I've done some professional singing." Singing had nothing to do with the job (or so I thought), but I figured if they knew I could get up in front of strangers and sing, they would hopefully believe I could do anything. As it turned out, they got very excited about this stating, "We have an employee band, and they are desperate for a singer." They now looked more enthusiastic and interested than they had throughout the entire interview. Needless to say, I was hired into a job that was pivotal in my life and career on many levels. To this day I'm sure that they hired me as much because I could sing as for my other capabilities. All that mattered to me was that I got the job. Had I not asked those critical questions, I would not likely have shared that information, and who knows what would have happened. But since I knew exactly where I stood going in there and what I was up against — in other words I was well prepared — I got creative in my approach, and it paid off big dividends.

Frequently Asked Questions About Interviewing

Q: *Should I accept coffee if offered to appear sociable?*

A: You should never eat or drink anything on a traditional interview (exception: interview over a meal or a drink in a public place) even if the interviewer is doing so. Remember this is not a social call. Besides, there is too much potential for disaster while wielding hot coffee.

Q: *Am I obligated to tell a prospective employer about a medical problem I have?*

A: According to the Americans with Disabilities Act, you are only obligated to mention a medical condition or disability if you will need special accommodation made on the job. We'll discuss special challenges related to disabilities in Chapter 9.

Q: *What if I decide during the interview that this is not the right job for me?*

A: Proceed with the interview anyway as if you were interested. As previously mentioned, there are many times that a different and often better job is offered afterwards. Also, the interview is an opportunity to establish a relationship with the employer, and you never know where that will lead now or in the future. Also, it's always a good idea to take a day to consider everything you learned about the job and to consider what's in it for you.

Q: *Should I carry a briefcase?*

A: It's better not to because then you have to worry about carting it around or accidentally leaving it somewhere. Besides, some prospective employers consider it overkill. If you want to carry some extra copies of your résumé, etc., use a professional looking folder or portfolio that is unobtrusive.

Q: *Is it OK to carry a small notebook and take notes?*

A: Yes, as previously noted, it is perfectly acceptable as long as you are not constantly writing. You want to stay engaged with the interviewer.

In Chapter 8 we'll continue our discussion about interviewing, including what to wear, interview follow-up, salary negotiation, accepting a job offer, and more.

Interviewing Two: The Sequel

Now that we've covered some interviewing basics, it's time to get more specific. Knowing how to respond to "special" questions, what to wear to an interview, how to handle various types of interviews, and how to properly follow up after an interview will make you feel more confident and in control. And if you use all the tips offered, you might find yourself in the enviable position of fielding job offers from several prospective employers. Then comes choosing the right offer, salary negotiation, and resigning from your current job. So, let's get started.

Other Types of Questions

In addition to the most commonly asked interview questions discussed in Chapter 7, some interviewers may also ask a variety of other types of questions. These range from more in-depth or situational questions to the abstract. Following are several different types of questions you may encounter along with tips on how to handle each.

Situational Questions

This category of questions, also known as behavioral questions, usually starts with the phrase, "What would you do if...?" or, "Tell me about a time that...." You're given a hypothetical situation or problem or are asked to relate a real experience, asked how you would or did handle it, or how you would or did solve the problem. This type of question is sometimes asked in a more general way by stating, "Tell me about a problem you once experienced at work and how you solved it?" It might also be more specific such as, "Tell me about a difficult patient or client you once had. How did you handle the situation?" Understand that the interviewer is attempting to ascertain how you handle problems when they come up. In other words, are you rationale, logical, and clear-thinking, or are you reactionary and defensive with a tendency to fly off the handle? Employers are wondering not only if prospective candidates have critical thinking skills, but does the candidate apply and use critical thinking.

• •
It's OK to think for a few seconds before answering.
• •

When asked this type of question, take a moment to compose your thoughts. Think in terms of what the interviewer is interested in hearing about. Keep your response simple, direct, and brief. Get right to the point and don't embellish. Remember the interviewer is looking for a logical thought process and a good outcome. Situational questions might also be used to evaluate a particular skill set. For example, "Tell me about a time

A nurse once wrote to me in a state of despair having just come back from an interview where she was completely thrown by a situational question. She told me that the interviewer said to her, "A coworker comes up to you in the hallway at work and starts screaming at you about something. What would you do?" She felt at a complete loss as to how to respond to this question and believed that she blew the interview as a result. She wanted to know how she should have answered this question for future reference.

I first reminded this nurse of why this type of question is asked and what the interviewer's objective is: to ascertain how she handles problems when they come up.

I suggested that an appropriate answer would be something like, "I would respond in a calm manner by saying something like, 'You're clearly upset and I would be happy to discuss this further with you. But let's take it into the conference room so we don't disturb any of the patients or visitors.' I'd then start to walk toward the conference room in a way that included the other person." That answer probably would have satisfied the interviewer.

that you had to plan a project or program at work or school. What were the steps involved and what was the outcome?"

When responding to a situational question about a real experience, you may want to employ what's known as the STAR method to keep your thoughts and your response organized and on target. STAR stands for —

Situation — Describe a situation or problem
Task — Discuss what needed to be done and why
Action — Tell what specific actions or steps you took
Results — Highlight outcomes, accomplishments, etc.

Abstract or "Creative" Questions

Some interviewers like to use indirect or more abstract questions that they believe will give them insight into the candidate's character or personality. Below are actual questions that nurses have been asked on job interviews along with suggested answers and tips. When choosing an answer to these and other abstract questions, remember to think in terms of what the employer is interested in hearing about. You might answer these questions differently if asked in a social situation. Stay focused on the purpose at hand.

Q: *What's your favorite book that you read in the last six months?*

A: As this is a job interview, choose a title of an appropriate book (no romance novels or politically controversial books please) you read recently or in the past. If you haven't read any books in the last six months, rather than revealing that, think of something you read in the past. Remember, the interviewer is trying to learn more about you, so saying, "I've been too busy to read," does not help your cause.

Q: *When you die, what do you want written on your tombstone?*

A: "Janet; she always got the job done." That one is sure to elicit a smile from the interviewer and a good feeling.

Q: *Imagine yourself getting an award — what award would it be?*

A: "Employee of the century."

Q: *Who do you admire most?*

A: A nurse once asked me how she should have answered this question on a recent interview. I responded by asking, How did you answer it? She said, "My mother. She always had a zest for life and an appreciation of the little things that made life worthwhile, even while raising three kids and holding down a job." I couldn't top that answer. You can't go wrong with Mom!

Q: *Leave me with one word to remember you by.*

A: Here are some good responses: Dedicated, Determined, Compassionate, Enthusiastic.

Additional tips: It's OK to think for a few seconds before answering this type of question. Compose your thoughts and then speak. Be as natural and relaxed as possible with your response. Try to think of an answer that best serves your cause or purpose. This is something you get better at with some practice.

Illegal Questions

It is illegal to ask job candidates questions related to their religion, nationality, race, sexual orientation, marital status, health status, whether or not you have children, etc. This, however, does not prevent some unscrupulous prospective employers from asking the questions anyway. Here are some suggestions on how to handle the questions if they are asked.

Example: An interviewer asks in a very friendly and nonchalant manner, "So, do you have kids?" Knowing this is an inappropriate question on an interview, you might reply in an even tone, "Does that have any bearing on the job?" You're letting the interviewer know, in a professional manner, that you don't intend to answer the question because you know it shouldn't be asked. They'll get the message and will hopefully move in another direction.

Beware of indirect questions meant to elicit the information without directly asking the question. For example, an interviewer might say, "I hate going to my kids' soccer games every weekend, how about you?" You could answer with a little humor and with a smile on your face by replying, "Are you asking if I hate to go to YOUR kids' soccer games, too? Will that be a requirement of the job?" It will create a light moment, and the interviewer will see that you are savvy and sharp and not to be messed with.

Fortunately, the majority of interviewers are well versed in the laws regarding hiring and interviewing and are professional and ethical when it comes to screening and interviewing a job candidate. However, there are always those who try to circumvent the law and want to see what they can get away with. I only encountered this behavior on one interview in my career. Not surprisingly, it became quickly apparent to me that I did not want to work for this individual. I finished up the interview, did not bother to send a follow-up note in this case, and moved on.

I once interviewed for a medical sales position with a small entrepreneurial company. I first met with one of the coowners of the company; all went well, and I was asked to meet the other owner. This second person was the scientific partner and clearly had less business sense overall. After our initial introduction and upon sitting down in his office, he began to frantically search his desk for my résumé. When it became apparent he wouldn't be able to readily find it, I pulled another copy out of my portfolio. He was visibly impressed at my preparedness. So far so good. Then, without looking up at me (he was "acting" as if he were focused on my résumé), he asked, "Are you married?" I paused for a moment, knowing this was an inappropriate question, but not having any experience with this sort of thing, took a brief moment to compose myself. I thought to myself, I have a wedding ring on my left hand so it would be easy to determine that I am married, so I decided to respond, "Yes. Are you?" purposefully diverting the attention back to the interviewer. He seemed flustered by my counter question and in a nervous twitter, responded, without ever looking at me, "Oh yes, I am." And then, without missing a beat, and still not making eye contact with me (I'm certain he knew that what he was doing was illegal and unethical), he then asked, "Do you have children?" Now I was getting miffed but didn't want to abruptly terminate the interview since I was rather interested in the position up to this point. So I took a deep breath and after a too long pause, replied, now in a rather curt tone of voice, "No, do you?" He replied that he did not either but still seemed unprepared for my counter question.

The interview deteriorated from there. The more time I spent with this person, the more I realized what an idiot he was. I knew I could never work for him or his company. So after the interview, I never bothered to send a follow-up note and never heard from them again, nor did they hear from me. The job, as I already knew, would involve some international travel. I'm sure this person was interested in my personal life to determine if he thought I'd be distracted or have split loyalties. Of course it was none of his business and had I been more experienced with this type of situation, I would have answered his questions in the way I suggest above, "Does that have anything to do with the job?"

If you're feeling nervous and rusty, get out and do some informational interviewing to feel more confident.

What to Wear to an Interview

Your overall appearance is a critical part of a job interview. As previously mentioned, first impressions are made in as little as three seconds, and once they are in place, they are powerful and lasting. So, what can someone tell about you in three seconds? They can get a sense about you based on your appearance, including your clothes, accessories, grooming, posture, eye contact, and facial expressions, etc. Countless studies have been done to indicate that each of us makes preliminary judgments and forms opinions about people based on overall appearance. That is why your appearance, including what you wear on a job interview, is so critical.

Remember: An interview is a formal business situation, not a casual meeting or a social call. Therefore you should look sharp, talk sharp, and act sharp. In any interview situation, even if you're not sure if you want the job, you want to be one of the best, if not the best candidate for any job. Not only do you want to be viewed in the best possible light on every level, but you want to position yourself to be considered for the best job available (not always the one you're applying for) and the best compensation right from the beginning.

The traditional conservative view for interview attire is that a woman wears a skirted business suit and a man a traditional business suit. Wearing a business suit to an interview shows a seriousness of purpose on your part, shows respect for the person you are interviewing with, and will make you feel more confident and look your professional best. Your clothes make a loud statement about who you are.

This does not mean that you will not be hired if you wear a dress or slacks or sports jacket and khaki pants. On the contrary, many people have interviewed in attire other than a business suit and been hired. But the better you dress, the more professionally and favorably you are viewed. While you may have heard that other attire is acceptable, a suit still makes the best impression. Besides, "acceptable" doesn't cut it in today's competitive job market. Even if you are of a younger generation and believe that casual dress is more the norm for your generation, you may be interviewed by someone from an older generation (a different age group) or simply someone who has a traditional view of interview attire. Conservative and traditional attire is a sure bet in most situations.

There are two exceptions to the business suit rule: If you are a woman who never wears skirts for whatever reason, then wear a pants suit. If you wear certain attire for religious reasons, that is acceptable.

What color should you wear? It is always best to stay conservative on an initial interview until you get a better feel for the company and their culture. Safe, conservative colors for both sexes are navy, grey, and black. Colors such as maroon or dark green are also acceptable for a woman. Avoid pastels. Red is considered an aggressive color, and while it would not typically be worn to an interview by a woman, I once wore a red suit to an interview for a sales position because I wanted to appear assertive and outgoing. It apparently worked because I was offered a job. Men should wear a white shirt and conservative tie.

Women should wear closed-toe pumps and hosiery (no bare legs) and men traditional oxfords and dark socks. Shoes should be polished and in good repair.

Your grooming should be impeccable. Hair should be neat and off your face. Keep your accessories simple and tasteful. Makeup, perfume, and cologne should be at a minimum. In fact you are better off avoiding scents, since some people are allergic or are turned off by certain scents.

If you smoke, avoid smoking for a while prior to an interview. If you have a cigarette just before walking into an interview, non-smokers can smell it immediately, and it is a turnoff to many people.

Interview Follow-Up

An important, but often ignored aspect of interview etiquette is sending a thank you or follow-up note after the interview. A note, which should be sent no later than the day after the interview, sets you apart from the other candidates. The note should be short and to the point. Thank the interviewer for the time spent, express your continued interest in the position, and briefly summarize what you would bring to the job. If more than one person interviewed you, send a note to each person. (Before you leave the interview, ask for business cards from each person who interviewed you.)

Your thank you note should be word-processed on good-quality stationery. Can the letter be handwritten? Although a few employers find it more personal, many consider a handwritten note unsophisticated. How about an e-mail thank you? That's only appropriate if you're applying to a technology company or have a short window of opportunity. For example, if you have a second interview with the same person the following day, a traditional thank you letter won't have time to reach its destination. In that case, an e-mail will serve the purpose. But of course, you can still send a traditional note to those whom you won't be seeing again. It's not necessary to send multiple thank you notes to the same person for subsequent interviews.

What if, after the interview, you've decided you don't want the job? Don't be so quick to walk away. Send the thank you note and proceed as if you wanted the job. There are many times that a different — often better — job is offered. Every interview is an opportunity. You never know what may happen. The better time to decline a job is when you're asked to interview again or are offered a position.

Then, if you haven't heard anything from the employer within the designated time as discussed in Chapter 7 (When might I expect to hear from you?), make a follow-up phone call to the person that interviewed you. Say something like, "Hello, Ms. Hawkins. My name is Carol Garfield. You may recall that I interviewed for the ICU staff position about two weeks ago. I was wondering if you had made a decision yet?" Since the interviewer has likely interviewed several people for the position, they may not immediately recognize your name so you might add something to jog their memory like, "I am the nurse that works in County General. You and I discussed so and so college while I was there."

If Ms. Hawkins says she's still interviewing for the position, then you should ask, even if you already asked this on the original interview, "Do you have any reservations about me that I can clear up while you have me on the phone?" Why ask now or why ask again? Let's face it: If you were the ideal candidate, you'd probably have been offered a position already. If you open the door, they may be honest. It gives you an additional opportunity to sell yourself and overcome any perceived objections. Just asking the question shows you're a motivated, assertive person who's obviously interested in the job. If any objections are expressed, use the strategies and responses suggested in Chapter 7.

On the other hand, if the interviewer has already filled the position, you might say, "I'm always working on my interview and self-marketing skills. I respect your opinion and wonder if you might give me some tips on how I might improve my presentation and marketability next time." Although it takes a bit of courage to ask this question, it can yield some invaluable feedback. Get something positive from the experience.

If you can't reach the interviewer by phone, you might try human resources or nurse recruitment to check on the status of the position. You can also try e-mailing the interviewer in this circumstance. Unfortunately, some employers don't get back to all the people they interview. If you remain unsuccessful in reaching the parties involved after multiple attempts, you may have to regroup and move on. That's why it's always good to have a few irons in the fire.

The Right Approach for the Right Interview

So far we've focused primarily on the traditional hiring interview. That's the type in which you meet face to face with the person for whom you'll likely be working directly. But there are actually many different types of interviews, and each presents its own challenges. Here are a few common types and some tips to get the most out of the experience.

The screening interview: This is a preliminary procedure usually conducted by someone other than the individual for whom you'd be working, most likely someone from human resources or a nurse recruiter. It might be done in-person or by telephone. The purpose of a screening interview is to make sure job candidates meet certain minimum standards. It's also an opportunity to weed through the applicants and eliminate those who don't seem to have the "right stuff," either by background or personality.

Because this is only a preliminary interview, you don't have to elaborate on all of your work experience and special skills. You should answer the interviewer's questions succinctly. There's no need to ramble or elaborate. Don't offer any additional information unless it's particularly relevant to the position. And while you don't have to give your whole sales pitch to this person — the hiring interview is still to come — you do have to impress the interviewer with your character, personality, attitude, and appearance if in-person. Be friendly, courteous, and professional every step of the way.

Technically, it's not necessary to send a thank you note after a screening interview, although it certainly doesn't hurt depending on the length and depth of the interview. It's an opportunity to express your interest in the job and demonstrate professionalism.

The phone interview: The telephone interview has become popular both as a screening tool and as a device to interview candidates at a distance. It presents a unique challenge for the job candidate because there's limited opportunity to convey strong nonverbal communication. The interviewer can't see you; he or she can only hear you.

Prepare for a phone interview beforehand just as you would a traditional interview. If this is other than a screening interview, write down some points you want to make and any questions you want to ask.

When the time for the interview arrives, be sure to go to a quiet location with minimal distractions where you're not likely to be disturbed.

Remember, the other party can hear what's going on in the background, so if a radio is playing, a baby is crying, you're shuffling papers around, hitting computer keys, or smoking a cigarette, the interviewer will be able to hear it. Telephone receivers are very sound sensitive.

When it's time to talk, put a smile on your face even though the person on the other end can't see it. When you smile, there's something in your voice that conveys friendliness and confidence. Use an enthusiastic and assertive tone, and listen attentively. Speak slowly and clearly, taking time to enunciate your words. And even though the interviewer can't see you, dress professionally for the interview; research has demonstrated that people act more professionally when they are dressed the part.

If the phone interview is something other than a preliminary screening interview, send a thank you note.

The follow-up interview: This is often one in a series of hiring interviews for a specific position. It might be done with the person who previously interviewed you or with different people. The purpose is to see how you fit in with the team and to get to know you better. Don't let down your guard or assume you have the job because you're being brought back: Dress and act as sharp as you did during the first interview. If possible, wear a different outfit for each visit. Be prepared for situational questions, such as, "What is the first thing you'd do as manager if you get this job?" or, "How would you handle this situation?"

Reminder: As discussed in Chapter 7, be sure to ask if anyone else is being brought in for a second interview, or if anyone else is also being considered for the position. If the answer is yes, ask, "Where do I stand with the competition?" Remember, it is often the best prepared candidate that gets the job.

Send a thank you note to anyone who interviewed you for the first time. While it is not necessary to send another typed note to the same person for subsequent interviews, this is one situation where a short e-mail follow-up is appropriate such as:

Dear Amad,

It was nice to see you again today. Thank you for setting up the interview with Allen and Fred. I enjoyed meeting them and further discussing the position. We certainly had some lively discussion! I look forward to our next meeting.

Best Wishes,
Ayesha

The panel interview: This is when you're interviewed by more than one person in the same room at the same time. This is sometimes done as the preliminary interview in a series, or it might be the format for a subsequent interview. The panel might be various members of a particular department, or it might be several supervisors or managers if you're applying for a management position. That's why it's important to always ask beforehand who will be interviewing you. Reminder: Get the names and titles of those involved. That way, you'll be well prepared.

A panel interview can be intimidating, but it doesn't have to be if you're prepared. On entering the interview room, make eye contact with all the participants and shake each person's hand before and after the interview, even if you have to walk around a table to do so. Listen carefully to each person's name and repeat it after it is told to you. This will help you to remember it when you first hear it. If possible, address everyone by name during the interview. (This is not absolutely necessary so don't panic.) However, it will win you some points if you can manage to do it. One person will likely take the lead during the interview and ask most of the questions, but be sure to direct your answers to and make eye contact with, everyone in the room. Ask for each person's business card at the end of the interview, shake everyone's hand again, tell them it was a pleasure to meet with them, and thank them for their time. Send a follow-up note to each person.

The in-house interview: This is an interview for another position than your current one with the organization that you already work for. For example, you might currently be a staff nurse in a hospital and have decided to apply for a unit manager position or staff development job. Treat this type of interview as you would any other, even if you are already acquainted with the person who will be interviewing you. That is, apply for the position using a cover letter and submitting a résumé.

When it's time for the interview, try to make the appointment before or after your work hours or on your day off so that you are not distracted and can be more focused. It is ideal if you wear proper interview attire to the interview even if you have to change at work. Send a thank you note and follow the described follow-up procedure.

The dinner interview: Interviews conducted over dinner are most common when applying for a management position, or one in which you will be dealing with the public, such as a sales or marketing position. It gives both parties an opportunity to get to know each other in a less structured format. It's also an opportunity for the interviewer to better observe your social graces, and your ability to handle yourself in a variety of situations.

To prepare, brush up on your dining etiquette beforehand, if necessary, by referring to appropriate books or articles. Follow the interviewers lead when ordering appetizer, entrée, etc. You don't have to order the same thing as them, but you should order something in the same general price range and of the same type. If the interviewer doesn't order an appetizer than you should forgo the appetizer as well.

Proceed with caution where alcoholic beverages are concerned. If the interviewer orders a glass of wine or beer, it would be appropriate for you to also order same — only if you wish — and only at a dinner interview (not at lunch). If you do order alcohol, stick to wine or beer (and *only* if the interviewer also orders the same) and sip your drink and don't finish it. If you don't want an alcoholic beverage, it's fine to order a soft drink or water. One recruiter I spoke with is of the mind that a job candidate should not order any alcohol on an interview. Use your best judgment and always err on the side of caution.

Remember that it's still an interview — not a night out — so dress and act accordingly.

The group interview: This is the type where multiple candidates are interviewed as a group, often at a facility open house or open application event as well as for graduate school applicants. You can stand out from the crowd by being appropriately dressed, by making good eye contact with the interviewer, and smiling as appropriate. Ask one or two questions when the opportunity presents itself, but don't dominate the session. Afterwards, be sure to approach the interviewer(s), introduce yourself and shake his or her hand. Obtain this person's business card, provide yours if you have one (you should!), and send a thank you note, even for a graduate school interview. All of this will help to distinguish you in a positive way.

The impromptu interview: This type of interview is conducted at career fairs or at on-site open house events. There is usually a crowd present and a fair amount of noise and activity. Both the recruiter and the prospect are standing and conversing. An impromptu interview is brief and preliminary to give the recruiter a sense of whom they wish to speak with further after the event. Make a good first impression by being well dressed and well prepared with your résumé and business card. Shake hands, make good eye contact, and smile. Present yourself as friendly, upbeat, personable, and enthusiastic. Since there is little time at these events to discuss specifics, convey interest in the employer's need, express your particular interests but remain open to further discussion and possible opportunities. In other words, keep an open mind. This approach is guaranteed to get you a call-back.

There are some occasions when recruiters at these events have made arrangements to have more in-depth interviews with candidates that they are interested in. So, if you make a good impression and have the background that the recruiter is looking for, you just might be asked to sit down somewhere to talk further. It happens sometimes, so be prepared!

The teleconference (video) interview: This type of interview allows both parties to see and interact with one another regardless of geographic location. Because special technology is required, teleconference interviews would most likely be conducted in the office of a professional recruiter, at a local branch of a company or facility that has other locations, from a college campus career office, or in an employment agency office.

Prepare as you would for any interview. Dress in subdued colors, avoiding red, white, stripes, and patterns since these do not show well on video and certain patterns can appear to "move" on camera. Wait for the other party to finish speaking completely before responding. Listen attentively, and use good nonverbal communication (sit upright, smile as appropriate, and make good "eye contact" with the camera). Focus on the recruiter's image and don't be distracted by your own image, usually shown on another screen or window. In this type of interview, hand gestures should be minimal since they can be distracting.

Juggling Job Offers

It's bound to happen at some point. You're going on multiple job interviews, trying to find just the right spot for your next career move. Things are going fairly well, and you've found several different positions that interest you. So far so good, right? But what if you get offered one job while waiting to hear from another that you prefer? Or what if you're offered a job before you've even interviewed for the position in which you're really interested? Learning professional strategies to juggle job offers will help you find the position that's right for you.

Scenario One: You've been on several interviews. Although all of the positions interest you, there's one in particular you're really excited about, and you hope you'll get an offer for it. In the meantime, you get an offer for another position. The pay is pretty good, and it's a good company. You can picture yourself working there, but you can't help but wonder about the other position. Should you say no to the offer and hold out for the position you really want? Or should you take the offer, knowing even though it may not be your ideal job, you'll feel more secure and can stop interviewing?

Strategy: There's a natural tendency to grab the first job offer that comes your way because it gives you a sense of security. However, the purpose of interviewing is to thoroughly explore your options and find a position that's a good move for you.

Tell the company that's making the offer you're interested in the position, but you're actively interviewing and need a little more time to consider your options. Some companies will take this better than others. You might ask, "May I have a few days to think it over?" Most employers are unwilling to wait very long for an answer. Understandably, they'll want to move on to the next candidate if you decide you don't want the job. They'll probably give you a time frame to respond or ask you how much time you need. Negotiate for as much time as possible, but be reasonable. No employer will wait forever while you make up your mind.

Then contact the employer you're really interested in working for. Tell the company you've received another job offer, but you'd prefer to work for them. Because you have to make a decision about the other job offer within a reasonable period of time, ask what your prospects are. Even if your ideal employer is not yet ready to make a final decision, it's hoped the company will be honest with you about your chances of getting hired. At least you'll know where you stand.

Scenario Two: You've met with some prospective employers and still have some interesting interviews lined up. One upcoming interview sounds particularly intriguing, and you're looking forward to learning more about the position and the company. Before the interview occurs, you receive a job offer from another company. The offer is tempting, but you're dying to take a shot at the other position.

Strategy: As in the first scenario, let the employer who made the offer know you're actively interviewing and would like a little more time to consider all of your options. Call your ideal employer and tell them you've received another job offer. Let them know you're particularly interested in the position they advertise and ask if the interview can be moved up. You can advise them you'd like to see if the job might be a good fit for both parties before you make a decision about the other offer. Of course, if that isn't possible, then you may have to take your chances and let the first job go while you pursue the other.

Scenario Three: Another possibility is you receive two or more job offerings within the span of several days. It has happened! One of the jobs offered is your distinct preference, but the other job offers better salary, benefits, hours, or whatever.

Strategy: See if you can buy some time from the offering employers. Tell your preferred employer that you're most interested in this position but have been made another offer with a better salary or benefits, etc. Ask if there is any room for negotiation. Stress that you would prefer to work for them and would be able to easily make your decision if the salary, benefits, etc., could be matched or at least improved. You're at an advantage here, but don't flaunt it. Be honest with your ideal employer, and see if you can work things out.

How to Negotiate the Salary You Want

Unfortunately, it's impossible to negotiate salary in every position you go after. For example, when you apply for a staff position in a public health-care facility, salaries are usually predetermined and pretty much set in stone. They're based on objective criteria, such as years of experience, degrees, certifications, shift differential, and so on. However, once you get into management, or in some cases, private healthcare facilities and more nontraditional jobs, there is usually leeway to negotiate.

Here are the rules for successful salary negotiating:

Do your homework. Find out what the going salary is for a comparable position in your geographic area. Search Internet job databases or contact the state arm of a related national professional association for salary surveys or information. For example, if you are applying for a nurse educator's position in a hospital, contact your state chapter of the National Nursing Staff Development Association and find out if the chapter or the national office has done any salary surveys in the last five years.

Another effective way to find salary information is to network with others in the industry. While it's considered rude to ask someone how much she or he makes, it's perfectly acceptable to ask, "What's a ballpark salary for a hospital-based nurse educator position in this geographic area?" If you can't find information on the same job in the same type of setting, look for something with similar responsibilities. This type of information can be obtained through routine informational interviewing, or you can simply conduct your own informal salary survey. In the later case, promise to share your findings with those who offer you information.

Let them mention a number first. Once you've been offered a job, try to get the prospective employer to quote a number or salary range first. In an employment situation, whoever mentions a salary figure first is at a disadvantage. So if you're asked what you think would be a fair salary, say something like, "How much have you budgeted for this position?" or, "How much were you paying the last person? Let's start there." Many employers will be up-front with this information. Then you can gauge what you have to work with.

Know your bottom line. Be prepared ahead of time with a ballpark amount that you want, based on your knowledge and experience. What's the least amount you're willing to take? And since both salary and benefits make up your total compensation package, you have to look at the big picture; don't fixate solely on hourly rate or annual wages. Consider the total healthcare coverage package; does it include eyeglass and dental coverage? How much tuition reimbursement is offered? Does the employer have a 401k program with matched annual savings? Are you eligible for a pension? Everything has an associated dollar value.

Likewise, you have to consider the general working conditions and schedule as well as the type of work you will be doing. For example, how much vacation is allotted? I once spoke with a nurse who took a $6,000/year pay cut when she transitioned from the hospital to a law office working as a legal nurse consultant. However, she received more comprehensive healthcare benefits for herself and her family, and she got seven weeks of paid vacation! That was worth more to her than the extra salary. Benefits can account for up to half of your total compensation package.

Ask for a little more money than you're offered. There's usually a salary range, and people rarely offer the top amount. If your request is reasonable and the employer wants you and has the budget, you may get what you ask for. The worst that could happen is that you get turned down. But asking doesn't jeopardize your standing unless you make a completely unrealistic request.

Be prepared to sell yourself. When offered an amount that is considerably less than you had hoped for, you might say after a slight pause, "I was hoping you would come in closer to (whatever amount you were hoping for or a little higher), based on the level of responsibility and skill required to do the job." Then you have some room to negotiate down, if necessary. If the money is there, then the negotiating begins. You can always come down with your salary requests, but you can't go up once you've stated a number. When you can't get the money you want, you can negotiate vacation time, tuition reimbursement, or other things that come out of a different budget.

Frequently Asked Questions

Q: *What if I'm offered a job on the spot?*

A: While this can be very flattering, it is always best to take some time to think over everything just discussed and be certain this is what you want. You could respond with "Wow, that is tempting. I would appreciate the opportunity to sleep on it before giving you my final answer." There is nothing wrong with this, and it shows you are intelligent and logical rather than impulsive or desperate!

Q: *Is it ever OK to ask for a tour of the department or the facility?*

A: Yes, under certain circumstances. Since prospective employers are usually interviewing multiple candidates, it may not be appropriate to ask for a department/facility tour on an initial interview. It would be very time consuming for an employer to bring every job candidate around. Of course if a tour is offered, accept. If you are brought back for a second interview that would be an appropriate time to ask for a tour.

Q: *What if I'm offered a job I don't want?*

A: If that happens, tell the employer that after considering everything, you have decided this is not the right position for you so you will have to decline. Thank them for their time and interest and wish them luck in their search. If they ask for more specifics as to why, you could say something like, (depending on the real reasons) "This is too much of a lateral move for me," or, "I realize I would prefer to do something more clinical in scope." If they say, "Is there anything we can do to change your mind?" If there is something, let them know. If not, say so.

Q: *What if I accept a job and then, for whatever reason, change my mind before I have actually started?*

A: While you should always accept a job in good faith after due consideration, you may still find yourself in this situation at one time or another. The important thing to do is to notify the prospective employer as soon as possible, ideally by telephone. If the person who interviewed you is not available, then speak to someone in human resources so that the message is conveyed immediately. It is not appropriate to send this type of message by e-mail or to leave a voice mail message; these forms of communication are unreliable and are too informal to convey such a message. It is never appropriate to simply not show up on your designated start date as a way of getting your message across. Remember, you never know when you'll run into the people who interviewed or hired you at another time in another location. Your behavior — good or bad — will follow you wherever you go.

Q: *What if they ask if they can contact my current employer?*

A: If you are job searching while employed elsewhere, the likelihood is that your current employer doesn't know you're looking nor would you want them to. Simply answer this question by saying, "No." That is perfectly normal and understood. It will not be held against you. In this circumstance, a recruiter may request a copy of the candidate's last performance evaluation, which has the evaluator's and candidate's signatures. This is another good reason why it's always good to request and retain copies of your performance evaluations.

Q: *What if my former company or facility has closed or been sold or moved? How do I explain that on a job application or reference check form?*

A: These things happen so just be straightforward about it. If the company is closed, you can list the employer but in the address section you can state, "Closed" or, "No longer in business." If the company/facility has been sold or acquired and now operates under a new name, list the name and address used when you worked there and add in parenthesis: (Currently known as "[current name if you know it]"). If a company relocated, and you have lost track of them, in the address section of an application you can note: Relocated. Current address unknown.

Q: *What if my former supervisors no longer work where I did? Who can I use as work references?*

A: For starters, your work references do not have to still work in the place where you worked with them, so that is not a problem. However, if an employer specifically wants to speak to a past supervisor or director from a particular job and that person no longer works there, you would simply tell that to the interviewer. This scenario is fairly common since so many people change jobs so often these days.

Q: *How much can/will a previous employer reveal about my past?*

A: Today, most employers are cautious about what they say about former employees. Some have a policy of only verifying titles and employment dates. That's not always the case with former supervisors. And remember, if you're applying for a patient care position, some states have laws regarding mandatory disclosure of certain information when requested by prospective healthcare employers related to clinical practice and patient care issues. We discussed how to deal with a problematic past in Chapter 7.

This is one reason why it is best to be honest and upfront about these situations if they exist in your employment history. If you conceal something like this and the employer finds out about it later, you will almost definitely be disqualified from the position. However, if you disclose the situation and address it adequately, the prospective employer may be willing to hire you in spite of it, depending on the situation.

When all is said and done, the majority of employers hire people (or don't) because of their personality. A positive, upbeat, can-do attitude is worth more to many employers than all the credentials and experience in the world.

Interviewing Essentials — A Review

- Be well prepared
- Be impeccably dressed and groomed
- Arrive early and take time to ground yourself
- Smile, make eye contact, and shake hands
- Be attentive, conversational, and ask questions
- Show interest in the job, the company, and the interviewer
- Every interviewer's style is different so go with flow
- Think in terms of what the interviewer is interested in
- Bring extra copies of your résumé and business cards
- Be courteous to everyone you encounter
- Let your personality shine through
- Turn negatives into positives
- Project a positive, upbeat, can-do attitude
- Act confident even if you don't feel confident
- End the interview on a positive note
- Send a thank you note within 24 hours
- Follow-up with a phone call if necessary

Choosing the Right Job for You

In deciding whether or not to accept a job offer, go back to the basics discussed in Chapter 3 about where to go from here. Reflect on what type of work you want to do, what you enjoy doing, what your ideal work environment and schedule would be like, and then contemplate how well this position meets those needs and interests. Consider how your lifestyle, including your family life, will be affected. Consider your commute, amount of paid vacation and personal time, and whether or not you would have to work holidays, weekends, or do shift work. Can you telecommute? Is the schedule flexible? What type of support staff is available to help you to do your job well? What is the dress code?

When all is said and done, the work and the company should provide an opportunity for you to learn and grow professionally. The work should be something that is interesting and even exciting to you. You should get paid a fair wage for your experience, credentials, and education. The schedule and workload should support your ability to have a good quality of life that includes time for your family and friends and your own self-care.

When accepting a job, ask to get the offer, including the salary and any special benefits discussed, in writing. Getting it in writing not only makes the offer official, but you have some documentation in case there is a discrepancy about what was agreed upon later. It has been known to happen. Look out for your own best interests.

How to Resign from Your Current Job

Once you've accepted a job and received the offer in writing, the first thing you must do if you're currently working elsewhere is notify your current boss. Don't tell anyone, other than your immediate family, about your new job until you have told your boss. Word gets around no matter how discreet you may be, and your boss should never hear about your resignation from someone else! I have seen it happen on more than one occasion. In fact, someone who once worked for me told her neighbor in a distant city about a new job she accepted. She was going to wait a few weeks before resigning because she wanted to collect some benefits that would accrue. The neighbor just happened to know a good friend of mine who mentioned it to her, not knowing it was supposed to be a secret. I of course heard about it and confronted my staff member. She was embarrassed beyond belief and did not leave on good terms as a result.

Every employer should have a policy related to resignation protocol, including how much notice must be given, so be sure to check that policy before doing anything. When notifying your current boss about your resignation, it is ideal to tell her/him in person. If you can't tell your boss in person in a timely manner, then resort to the telephone. This should be followed-up in writing immediately. It is always a good idea to give one copy to your boss and another to human resources. This way, no one can claim they didn't know, or that you didn't give proper notice. In other words, cover all your bases.

When writing your letter of resignation (see sample) and when informing your boss that you are leaving, it is best to stay professional with your words and your demeanor, regardless of the reasons that you are leaving. In other words, don't burn your professional bridges; it will never serve you well in life. Even if you don't like your job, your boss, or the company you work for, always write a professional letter of resignation. The purpose of the letter is to notify your employer that you are resigning. It is not the place to air your grievances. This letter will become part of your permanent record.

Some employers will conduct an exit interview with all employees before they leave. The purpose of this session is to learn more about why you're leaving and what, if anything, the employer could have done to keep you onboard. This information can be helpful to the employer for future recruitment and retention efforts. It can also help them to address internal problems if applicable. This is not a gripe session. Nor is it an opportunity to disparage someone you didn't get along with. However, if you are leaving because of unresolved problems or other issues such as short staffing or a hostile workplace, be constructive and professional in your remarks.

Another reason to leave on professional terms: You never know who might be sitting behind the desk five years from now at another company/facility when you go on an interview. Also, people know people who know other people, and your actions will have a ripple effect whether positive or negative. The choice is yours.

In Chapter 9 we'll discuss some additional job hunting and career challenges as well as advice and information for some unique and special situations in nursing, including various phases of a nurse's career.

Sample Thank You Letter
JANICE SMITH, RN
45 Lane Avenue
Smithville, New Jersey 00090
908-555-2222 Cell: 908-555-8686
jsmith@net.net

November 11, 20__

Mary Harris, RN
Director of Quality Management
Allenwood Hospital
311 City Street
Allenwood, New Jersey 22536

Dear Ms. Harris,

It was a pleasure meeting and speaking with you today. I am convinced that the position of Quality Assurance Coordinator at Allenwood Hospital is the right job for me and that I can contribute substantially to the department and the facility.

My strong clinical background combined with my excellent communication skills will allow me to do the job that needs to be done. Also, I am reliable, detail-oriented, and motivated to succeed.

If I can provide you with any additional information, please do not hesitate to contact me. Thank you for your time, and I look forward to speaking with you again soon.

Sincerely,

Janice Smith, RN

Janice Smith, RN

Sample Resignation Letter
JANICE SMITH, RN
45 Lane Avenue
Smithville, New Jersey 00090
908-555-2222 Cell: 908-555-8686
jsmith@net.net

November 11, 20___

Mary Harris, RN
Director of Quality Management
Allenwood Hospital
311 City Street
Allenwood, New Jersey 22536

Dear Ms. Harris,

Per our conversation earlier today, I am resigning my position as staff nurse effective December 11, 20___. I have accepted a position as a utilization review nurse with Health International.

I have enjoyed working at Allenwood Hospital and thank you for the opportunities afforded me.

Best of luck to you. I hope our paths cross again in the future.

Sincerely,

Janice Smith, RN

Janice Smith, RN

Special Situations and Career Challenges

Now that we've covered general job search and career management strategies, it's time to address specific situations and challenges that may occur at one time or another over the course of a nurse's career.

Job Hunting Challeges

So far, we addressed what to do when you go on an interview and accept a job offer. But what if your job search isn't going as well as you'd like? Maybe you're not getting any interviews, or you're getting interviews but not getting any job offers. Here are some common challenges related to job hunting along with strategies to overcome them.

Challenge #1: You're sending out résumés but not getting responses.

This could be happening for several reasons. Here are a few possibilities along with recommended solutions.

a. Your résumé and cover letter may be working against you. Look them over and ask yourself, Are they as good as they could be? Are they written in a current up-to-date format that showcases your unique experiences and presents you and your background in a positive light? Review résumé writing and cover letter basics in chapters 5 and 6. Ask someone who hires or coaches nurses to look at your résumé and cover letter and give you some feedback.

b. You could be using the wrong approach to job finding for the type of position you're going after or the industry you want to get into; take another tack. Network more, do informational interviewing, consider part-time or temporary work to break into the field or gain experience. Consider volunteering as a way to get your foot in the door somewhere.

Challenge #2: You're going on interviews but not getting any offers.

Remember, there is a lot of competition out there, especially for the good jobs. Consider the following strategies to increase your chances of getting a job offer.

a. Review interview basics in chapters 7 and 8. Are you doing everything you could be doing, as well as you can? Are you dressing appropriately? Are you able to answer usual questions and market yourself well? Are you able to articulate your strengths and assets? Are you following up as recommended in Chapter 8? Be honest in your self-assessment and work on improving your image, your technique, and your form. Use a career coach if necessary.

b. If you interviewed with someone you felt comfortable with, call them shortly after you find out you did not get the job. Tell them that you are working on perfecting your interview skills, that you respect their opinion as a professional, and that you were wondering if they could give you any suggestions on how you might improve your performance in the future. You would, of course, say this in a very friendly, nonchalant way, so the interviewer does not feel put on the spot to explain why they didn't hire you. Many people will respect this and give you some constructive feedback. Everyone I know who has ever done this tells me that while it is difficult to do, and sometimes difficult to hear, it is some of the most valuable feedback they have ever gotten. Remember, if what you are doing isn't working, then it's time to take a new approach.

Frequently Asked Questions

Q: *What if I never hear back from the interviewer after an interview?*

A: You should follow-up after any interview with a thank you note and a phone call or e-mail if necessary as described in Chapter 8. In some cases you may need to make several attempts to contact someone from the company (the person(s) who interviewed you and/or someone in human resources) to see what your status is. Unfortunately, there are times that an employer just never gets back to candidates. So if, after repeated attempts at follow-up, you still haven't gotten anywhere, you may need to just move on.

Q: *If I send in a résumé and don't hear anything, can I call to see if they received it?*

A: If a week or two has passed, and you haven't heard anything, it is appropriate to call to be sure your résumé was received. However, if you respond to a classified ad that does not identify the employer or provide a phone number, then you have little recourse for follow-up.

Assimilating into a New Position, Workplace, or Specialty

Whether you're thinking about changing jobs, getting ready to move into a new role, or returning to the workforce, it will be necessary for you to learn new things, meet new people, and step out of your comfort zone. In Chapter 3 we discussed challenges to moving forward that included coping with fear, risk avoidance, indecision, and excuse making. Be sure to reread that section whenever you are in the midst of change in your career. That being said, the following are practical strategies to help you make a successful transition in a variety of situations.

Changing Specialties

In Chapter 3 we discussed how to research various specialties and positions before making a decision to move. Once you've made that decision and have landed a job, it's important to take steps to acclimate yourself to your new specialty.

Strategies that work:

1. Immediately join and get active in a related professional association such as the Emergency Nurses Association (www.ena.org), or Academy of Medical-Surgical Nurses (www.medsurgnurse.org), or the American Holistic Nurses Association (www.ahna.org). You'll immediately start to get the association publications, and you'll be able to access Members Only sections of their websites. Some associations even provide online mentoring or chat rooms where you can tap into the wisdom of nurses experienced in any specialty. This will significantly increase your learning curve.

2. Get out to local chapter meetings of your specialty association, as well as state and national conventions and conferences. Go by yourself or ask your new coworkers who belong if you can tag along with them. You'll benefit from the education, information exchange, support, and networking at these events. Remember that while no one has "extra time" to network, networking will actually energize you and support your career in many ways.

You may be able to deduct all or part of your professional development expenses and fees, including travel expenses, dues, and book purchase price, so check with your accountant.

3. Find out what books and other resources exist related to your new specialty. Do an online book and article search, check with the related professional association, and ask others who work in the specialty for recommendations. Immerse yourself in self-study. Don't rely on your employer to provide all of your education and training. Become an expert on your own.

It's always scary to move in a new direction with your career, especially when you've developed some expertise in another area. While some nurses may consider changing specialties as "starting over again," that is hardly the case. Sure you'll have things to learn in your new setting, but you'll be expanding your knowledge base and experience and building on what you already know rather than starting from scratch. It's all in how you look at it.

Transitioning from Traditional to Nontraditional Nursing Roles

When making a transition from a traditional patient care position to something less traditional, such as case management, telephone triage, or legal nurse consulting, it is common for some nurses to feel uneasy. I've heard nurses refer to this as "changing careers," or "leaving nursing," neither of which is the case. The truth is that, as outlined in Chapter 1, nurses are versatile and multitalented. We are healers, teachers, and nurturers. There are many ways and places to make a difference — some direct and some indirect. We are vital at the bedside, but we are just as vital in every other aspect of the healthcare arena.

Is a nurse who works for an insurance company or who is an editor of a nursing magazine or who is a recruiter for a hospital or who does research any less a nurse than one who delivers direct patient care? Not at all. Actually, the more places we work, the greater impact we will have as healthcare experts and as patient advocates, the more we will get noticed and taken seriously, and the louder our collective voice will be. Besides, having options is a good thing. Just knowing you have options lessens your anxiety about the future.

When moving into a nontraditional role, not only will you have things to learn about your new specialty, but you may also be working in a different type of environment and be required to learn different types of skills. You may even be required to dress differently than you are accustomed to, e.g., business clothes vs. uniforms or scrubs. Because of this, many nurses when making such a transition will say, "I feel like a fish out of water." That feeling is normal and will dissipate as time goes on. Unfortunately, some nurses jump ship and return to their old jobs before giving themselves an opportunity to become comfortable in their new setting. Every new job, specialty, and work setting requires a period of adjustment. You have to set small, short-term goals for yourself and track your progress. Remind yourself that you are expanding your horizons and your experience base every day. Also, expand your view of who you are, what you do, and what you are capable of doing as a nurse.

Going from Expert to Novice

One fear particular to nurses in the process of making changes in their professional life is the fear of going from expert to novice. Many nurses have worked in a particular specialty, and in some cases, even for the same employer, for many years. They can handle everything that comes up. They know the language, the routine, and the people. They know how to answer all the questions that come up, and that's a very comfortable place to be. Then, when they consider advancing in their position, changing specialties or employers, or moving in a completely new direction like entrepreneurship or teaching, they will have a lot to learn and may feel like a novice for a time. The security of "knowing it all" is gone.

Here are a few helpful things to remember when making a change in your career:

1. Nurses have above average intelligence. What do I base this on? The fact that you made it though a strenuous educational program, passed a rigorous state licensing exam, and worked in the complex and ever changing world of healthcare.

2. Whether you realize it or not, you've constantly had to learn new things and been thrown into situations where you weren't always sure of yourself. You'll apply those same skills and abilities to any new practice setting you go after. And the way I look at it, you've already learned the hardest stuff in nursing school and in your first nursing job. Anything else is simply an expansion of what you already know and already do.

3. You only have to do something for the first time once. After you've done something even one time, you immediately start to gain experience.

• •

When I was a kid, I took swimming lessons at a local high school. After mastering some basics strokes, it was time to jump off the diving board into the deep end of the pool in order to advance to the next level. I had only swum in three-foot deep water so far and was scared to death to jump into water over my head — so much so that I considered dropping out of swimming.

And yet, as scared as I was, my desire to advance in the swimming program was strong. So I devised a plan — such as it was — to get me through. When the big day came, I decided I would walk to the edge of the board quickly, close my eyes, hold my nose, jump in, and pray that I wouldn't drown. It was one of the hardest and scariest things I ever did in my life. By some miracle, I survived the impact, came to the surface, and swam to the edge of the pool. Frightening as it was, the whole thing wasn't nearly as bad as I had anticipated. Isn't that always the way? Our fears are usually greater than the reality of a situation. I now had some "experience" under my belt. My second jump was a little easier and the third jump easier still because I knew what to expect and was a little better prepared. Before I knew it, the diving board became fun.

This was a great lesson for me — one that I still carry with me. To this day, whenever I have something scary to do for the first time, in my mind I walk quickly to the edge of the board, close my eyes, hold my nose, jump in, and pray. Whatever I have to face in life, using this mental technique, I always manage to "survive the impact, come to the surface, and swim to the side of the pool." Things always get easier after that.

• •

4. It only takes three to six months to master a new skill. So when you start something new, you have to set small goals for yourself. Tell yourself, OK, in three months I'm going to have a grip on the situation; in six months I'll be working pretty independently, and in one year it will be as if I've always been here. Keep in mind that each day on a new job or in a new role, you become more experienced than you were the day before.

Additional Strategies

In addition to learning about your new specialty or practice area when making any career change, it is important to take steps to assimilate into your new work environment. This involves getting to know staff members, becoming part of the team, understanding the corporate culture, and learning about systems, procedures, and equipment. I write extensively about these things in my book *Your First Year as a Nurse — Making the Transition From Total Novice to Successful Professional.* Although the book was written for new graduate nurses, sometimes it is helpful to go back to basics when making transitions. And since some of us never learned the basics to begin with, a review may provide some valuable information for being successful in your career at any phase.

To summarize, here are some key points included in *Your First Year as a Nurse:* Go out of your way to introduce yourself to staff members in all departments and on all shifts. Learn and use people's names. Greet people when you arrive to work each day and say good-bye at the end of the work-day. Participate in work-related social events. Make an effort to get to know your coworkers by having lunch with different people occasionally and just by showing interest in them. Be willing to learn from all of your experi-enced coworkers regardless of their title or position. Treat everyone with respect and be willing to help out as needed even if something is "not your job." Don't be afraid to ask questions or ask for help when you need it.

Going Into Advanced Practice

There are more and more nurses going into advanced practice (i.e., nurse practitioner, clinical nurse specialist, certified nurse midwife, certi-fied registered nurse anesthetist) these days for a variety of reasons. Of those who complete the requirements, many are very successful yet some never manage to get a foothold in their new role. This has less to do with the job market since advanced practice nurses (APNs) are working in an increasing number of roles and settings. It has more to do with APNs' abili-ty to market and promote themselves — something many nurses find diffi-cult to do.

Once you've elevated your degree, your certifications, and your level of practice, you also have to elevate your image, your expectations, your social skills, and your career management expertise. Also, you need to develop an expanded view of your new role in healthcare. Many APNs are still staff nurses at heart and haven't fully taken ownership of their new level of prac-tice. They aren't able to see themselves in a new role. This can become a bigger obstacle than you might imagine.

I often hear new APNs say, "I have no experience," or, "I'm just starting out." On the contrary, you already have many years of nursing experience (unless you are an APN entry to practice). You are simply expanding your experience and practice; not starting from scratch. You are taking your practice to the next level — not starting from square one. This is an important distinction to make.

Consider these strategies to make the most of your advanced practice status:

1. Polish your professional image. Have business cards made with your new credentials, dress well, and master assertive body language. Pay attention to the social graces, including using a full firm handshake in workplace or business and social settings. Remember, you can act confident even if you don't feel confident. You have to inspire confidence in others.

2. Build a support system of peers. Create a network of APNs for support, information exchange, and networking. One way to do this is to join and get active in your specialty association as well as a related advanced practice association. This means getting out to occasional meetings, conferences, conventions, and special programs. It may also mean getting on committees, running for office in the association, or working on special projects. It is critical to stay connected to your peers at this level of practice. Look for role models and mentors for inspiration, information, encouragement, and support.

3. Develop a new job finding strategy. Don't rely on traditional methods to find jobs such as classified ads. Most advanced practice positions are filled through networking or word of mouth. That means you have to get on the phone with all of your professional colleagues — physicians, nurses, administrators, and anyone else you know in the industry. Let them know of your new credentials and tell them what you're looking for. Ask for advice, when appropriate, and for referrals. For every one APN who has ever told me that the market is flooded with APNs, I can tell you about two prospective employers or colleagues who told me they are looking for an APN and can't find one.

Get in the habit of introducing yourself with your new credentials to others in workplace and social situations. You never know who you'll meet where. As mentioned throughout this book, the power of networking is far reaching. Besides, when you meet people and tell them you're an APN, that's a great opportunity for them to ask you questions about your role to promote understanding and acceptance of APNs.

4. Consider alternate practice settings. Look into opportunities in community health centers, clinics, collaborative practice with other physicians and APNs, and even self-employment. While traditional hospital employment may be what you are accustomed to, it's time to broaden your horizons and consider all of your options. Not only will this expand your opportunities, it may lead to more money, flexibility, and autonomy.

Do some informational interviewing with seasoned APNs to learn from their experience. Attend seminars and read books on self-employment, contract negotiation, and related professional issues. In other words, learn about the "business" of being an APN.

5. Learn to sell yourself. Rather than looking for an "opening" to fill, you may have to sell your new credentials to an employer or organization and actually create your own position and job description. You might also have to sell your role when an employer is looking for another type of professional. I know more than one APN who applied for a position when the employer was looking for a physician assistant. In each case the APN was able to convince the employer that an APN added more value to the position and would be a better choice. Don't expect all employers to suddenly understand your role in healthcare and automatically create positions for you. APNs are still an unknown and underutilized group in many ways. Self-promotion is key.

Once you land a job, enter into a collaborative practice, or start a business, continue to promote your role. Do this by creating brochures or fact sheets about what APNs do. Talk to colleagues and coworkers about your role and how they can best utilize your specialized knowledge and expertise. Explain to patients, in language they can understand, what it means to be an APN and what your role is — how you will be working with them and how you can help them. Just because you exist and have a spiffy new credential and title, it does not mean that those around you will automatically know what to do with you or understand your unique role. Self-promotion is self-preservation for the individual and the practice level.

6. Work on your communication skills. Read books and take courses in effective oral and written communication. This includes conversational communication, writing for business (letters, memos, proposals), public speaking, and writing for publication. As an APN you will be communicating with a broader range of people on a broader range of topics. It is imperative that you develop excellent communication skills on every level.

Also, it is imperative that you develop your professional practice and expand your sphere of influence through professional speaking and writing. Public speaking and writing for publication not only boost your credibility and visibility, they also help to position you as an expert as well as showcase the role and expertise of all APNs. And, of course, they allow you to reach more people with your specialized knowledge and have a greater impact. Don't restrict your writing and speaking to other nurses; target consumer audiences, physician groups, and other healthcare professionals.

Moving Into Management

If you aspire to get into a management position, take these positive steps.

1. Work on your education. An advanced degree will make you well rounded; more knowledgeable about systems, theory, and practice; and more marketable. It will also increase your confidence.

2. Join a related management association. The American Organization of Nurse Executives (www.aone.org) is open to all nurses regardless of their role or level of experience. Here you'll find role models, mentors, support, and education. Get active in your local chapter. The National Association Directors of Nursing Administration/Long Term Care (www.nadona.org) is open to all nurses who work in long-term care. The American College of Healthcare Executives (www.ache.org) requires a minimum of a bachelor's degree and a commitment to the profession of healthcare management for membership.

3. Seek out related assignments at work. Look for those that will help you to build related skills, such as working on the budget, schedule, policies, and procedures, etc. Get active on committees and special projects. All of these things will propel you forward in your career, make you more visible in your workplace, and build your confidence as well as your skill set.

4. Let your supervisor, manager, or director know about your aspirations. A good manager will support you in your goals by providing related learning experiences and considering or recommending you for positions when they come up.

Once you have a management position, even a supervisor's role...

1. Immerse yourself in self-study. Read and take courses related to the management of people in general as well as nursing and healthcare management. Just because you have the title or the responsibility doesn't mean you automatically become an effective leader. Management is not a skill you learn by experience alone. And you cannot rely exclusively on your employer to provide all of the support and education you need to be successful in your new role.

2. Seek role models and mentors. Look for individuals both at work, and through your professional associations to model yourself after and for support and advice. If you haven't already joined AONE, NADONA, or ACHE, what are you waiting for? You should also belong to your state nurses association and specialty association. Remember: No one succeeds alone. Besides, this is the best way to stay on the cutting edge with knowledge and information about your specialty, about trends in nursing and healthcare, and about effective management techniques and tools.

3. Work on professional development skill building. In addition to continuously developing your clinical and managerial skills, work on your communication skills, professional image, conflict management, and nego-tiation skills. All of these are necessary to be an effective leader. You set the tone for your department. You set the example. You must model the behav-ior you want to see in your staff. It is a big responsibility; take it seriously.

Phases of a Nurse's Career

There are various stages in nurses' careers, where our needs, our inter-ests, and our experiences are different. Here are some tips to help you suc-cessfully navigate through the most common phases.

Student Nurse

Nursing is the toughest job you'll ever love. In addition to your formal education and training while a student nurse, there are many additional things that you can do to prepare for your future career and give yourself a competitive edge. Here are several:

Make the most of your classes and clinical time. Show up and partici-pate. Do your own research and reading, ask questions, and ask for help when you need it. This is a special time to learn from experienced nurses — your instructors — and get all the nurturing and guidance you can.

Join and get active in the National Student Nurses' Association (www.nsna.org). Joining NSNA has many tangible benefits. For starters, you will receive publications targeted to student nurses with pertinent arti-cles, insights, book reviews, and more. You'll stay abreast of upcoming con-ventions and special programs. Many schools will allow students time off to attend these conventions. Also, membership looks good on your résumé and will make you more marketable. There are many leadership opportuni-ties within the association that you may wish to take advantage of. I know of one hospital system that markets specifically to NSNA members because they are viewed as the cream of the crop.

Consider part-time work in healthcare. The more clinical experience and exposure that you get during your student years, the more comfortable and confident you will feel upon graduation. You will also significantly increase your learning curve. So if your schedule allows it and your school permits it, look for work as a nurse's aide, patient care technician, emergency room technician, emergency medical technician (EMT), and so on. Some of these positions require specific training and certification courses, but others do not.

Some healthcare facilities offer student externships, which are paying jobs often offered in the summer months, specifically for student nurses. These programs have more structure and support and allow you to work with experienced nurses in various specialties. You will often have an opportunity to do even more during an externship than you might in a regular job as an aide or technician.

It is ideal to seek work, including externships, in a facility where you may wish to work after graduation. This will allow you to become familiar with the physical plant as well as many of the people and procedures. And while this does not guarantee that the facility will hire you afterwards, it certainly can't hurt, especially if you have made a good impression.

Consider volunteering: Volunteering is also an excellent way to gain experience, make valuable contacts, and find ongoing support for your budding nursing career from experienced, competent, and enthusiastic nursing professionals. Consider offering to help out at health fairs provided by your local department of health or by a local healthcare organization. Contact organizations such as the American Red Cross, American Heart Association, or other social service agencies of interest to you about volunteer opportunities. Look into opportunities in hospice care, adult day care, long-term care, etc.

Get out and network: Networking is a great way to make valuable contacts, learn about student and graduate nurse opportunities, and to find mentors and role models. Whenever possible, attend nursing conventions, conferences, career fairs, etc. Fortunately, most schools of nursing encourage and support these activities; take advantage of them. Be sure to bring business cards and résumés along!

Join a specialty association: If you happen to have a special interest in obstetrics, perioperative or emergency nursing, or others, join the related specialty association as a student member. Most nursing associations have such a membership category and the dues are nominal. This will provide an opportunity to learn more about the specialty, gain access to experienced members of the specialty and to members only areas of the website if applicable. It will increase your learning curve and give you a competitive edge if you decide to enter that specialty upon graduation.

New Graduate Nurses

Between graduation and licensing, there is that unique time of relief, anticipation, dread, fear, and celebration. It is a time of transition between student and licensed nurse. There are many things you can do during this time to facilitate a smooth transition.

Celebrate! Once you've graduated, take time to revel in your accomplishment and do something special to celebrate. Take some time off, if possible, to destress and bask in the glow of your accomplishment. Reward yourself in a constructive way for all of your hard work with a vacation, spa day, favorite activity, or time with friends and family.

Prepare for your licensing exam: To prepare for taking your licensing exam, it can be helpful to use some review books to acquaint yourself with the types of questions that will be asked. You can find NCLEX review books in your school library, the public library, and in bookstores. You can even find some free resources on the Internet. Some new graduates benefit from a more intensive review offered by education companies by way of live classes or educational materials such as CD-ROMs and review books. Review as necessary but don't over study. At this point you either know the material, or you don't.

In addition to material review, be sure to study strategies for successful test taking. Going through sample test questions helps to familiarize you with the process and get into the exam groove. It's important to remember that licensing exams test basic knowledge; they are not designed to trick or deceive. Just before the test, take time to destress and relax so you'll be well rested and focused. Use positive visualization — imagine yourself acing the test and passing with flying colors.

Get connected: If you want a successful career in nursing, you must immerse yourself in the community of nursing. Staying isolated will lead to unhappiness and a feeling of being overwhelmed, and will pave the road to

A certain percentage of new graduates don't pass NCLEX the first time. If it happens to you, don't despair. It's happened to more people than you might imagine. Once you get your license, no one will know how many times you took the test before passing. Go through the above steps again, this time with even greater resolve. Be sure to think positively. Picture yourself as a licensed nurse looking back on this time in your early career.

burnout. Once you are a licensed nurse, join and get active in your state nurses association. Once you've secured your first job, also join a related specialty association if you're not already a member, such as the American Association of Critical-Care Nurses (www.aacn.org). Tap into the wonderful support and resources that already exist in nursing rather than trying to go it alone. As a reminder, some associations offer online and other forms of mentoring to new graduates. Utilize everything that is available to you!

Choosing your first job: In choosing your first job, look for a facility that offers a long and comprehensive new graduate orientation program complete with preceptor, ideally six months in length or longer. Some facilities also offer mentors, in addition to preceptors. Mentors are usually nurses who you do not work with on a daily basis but who will meet with you to discuss how things are going and advise and support you in various ways.

If you have an interest in working in a particular specialty such as trauma, intensive care, psych, etc., find out if that specialty is available to new graduates at that facility and what type of specialty internship or specialized training is provided. I'm often asked, "Is it necessary to do two years of med/surg nursing before going into a specialty?" While med/surg is a good place for some nurses to start, it is not right for every nurse. There is no one right path for all nurses to follow. Every nurse must follow his heart and carve out his own career path.

If you're not sure what you want to do, consider starting out on a med/surg or telemetry floor where you'll be exposed to many different types of patients and procedures. If you're offered a position in a particular specialty simply because an opening exits on that floor, research the specialty and the unit before making a commitment. Sometimes fate steps in and makes up your mind for you by presenting an opportunity you might not have otherwise considered.

Keep in mind that while salary is important to everyone, it should not be a primary factor in choosing your first job. What is most important is that you find a position in a facility that will best support your role as a new graduate nurse and nurture your growth and development. This is a pivotal time in your career. Your first job will help lay the foundation for the rest of your career.

Once working: Keep in mind that nursing school was phase one of your education. Your first job as a licensed nurse is phase two. You still have much to learn and are not expected to know everything or do everything. Seasoned nurses will tell you that it takes a full year before you start to feel some level of confidence. It will take another year before you begin to develop some level of competency. Don't be discouraged. You'll be moving forward the entire time and gaining confidence and experience. And believe me, the destination is worth the journey. Here are a few tips to help you along the way:

- **Align yourself with friendly, competent nurses.** They are all over if you only look for them. Contrary to what you may have heard, the vast majority of nurses are supportive, professional, and happy to help and guide you.

- **Be proactive with your training.** Don't wait for someone to show you how to do something. Ask to observe, assist, or perform a procedure with an experienced nurse when the opportunity arises. Seek opportunities to learn.

- **Watch, listen, and learn.** Read policy and procedure manuals and utilize other resources on your unit. Ask questions when you need to. Learn from your experienced coworkers regardless of their title or position. An experienced tech, aide, or unit clerk has a lot of knowledge to share and can teach you tricks of the trade.

- **Offer to help others.** Even though you are inexperienced, you can help to turn or transport a patient, get supplies if needed, make a bed, etc. When you extend yourself to others, they will reciprocate.

- **Respect everyone you work with.** Always say thank you when someone helps you. Everyone is on the same team and each person plays a vital role.

- **Work on staying positive and focused.** It's easy to get down when you feel challenged and overwhelmed. Keep a journal, use motivational tapes and books, and keep a record of your progress and accomplishments. Record positive things that patients, staff, and family members say to you and make note how you are making a difference.

- **Advocate for yourself.** If you don't get along with your preceptor, speak to your manager or the nurse responsible for your orientation. If you're not getting enough exposure to different types of procedures or cases, ask for additional opportunities.

- **Immerse yourself in the community of nursing.** Join and get active in your state nurses association and specialty association. Create alliances, build support, and get connected. Staying isolated serves no useful purpose.

The Second Career New Graduate

Many nurses are coming to the profession later in life (not right out of high school), possibly as a second, third, or fourth career. It could be a homemaker in her 50s or 60s who never had a career outside of the home. It could be a 40-year-old woman with an MBA and 15 years of management experience in the business world. It could be a 60 or older year old man who owned a business for most of his life and is looking for something meaningful to do in his "retirement." It could also be a 30-something year-old man who has been working in another industry, such as the computer industry and is looking for a career where he can make a real contribution while making a good salary and benefits with opportunities for advancement.

The truth is that new nurses have such diverse backgrounds these days, and every employer has not adapted well to that diversity. Don't be surprised if some of your managers don't seem to know how to react to you because you have more management experience than they do, or if people assume you're experienced or that you're ready to retire because of your age. Take it all with a grain of salt and focus on the task at hand — honing your nursing knowledge and skills.

• •

Focus on your great skills and abilities and the contributions you can make.

• •

If you come from a business or corporate background, you will likely find the healthcare culture to be very different in a variety of ways, so be prepared. Although every place of employment is different, you may experience remnants of the old patriarchal days of healthcare when physicians ruled. You may find some new graduate nurse training programs to be geared toward the young, inexperienced learner. You may also encounter some nurses "from the old school" who believe that nurses should stay separate and not participate in facility-wide events, committees, or boards.

When the time feels right, after you've gained some nursing experience and have assimilated well into your new unit, offer to work on some projects or develop some educational programs where you can utilize skills, specialized knowledge, and talents that you acquired outside of nursing. Second-career nurses bring a broad range of unique skills, experiences, and credentials to nursing that have the potential to enrich and expand the profession in many ways.

Older Nurses

Let's face it, most of us are living and working longer. Retirement is being redefined and some have suggested that the word may be phased out of our vocabulary. That doesn't mean we can't kick back and slow down a bit in our older years — if we choose to do so. The truth is that many of us want to remain in the workforce in some capacity. Fortunately, the industry we work in recognizes and values that experience and maturity and is taking steps to accommodate us as we age.

Strategies for Older Nurses in the Workforce

That being said, some older nurses feel a bit insecure about their advanced age and are uncertain about their marketability at this stage in life. Also, age-related prejudice does exist in our society. Here are some tips to keep you connected, confident, marketable, and competitive.

Be confident in your experience. You've accumulated a great body of life and work experience that younger people don't have. Share it, but stay open to new ideas. In other words, be willing to be both teacher and student.

Develop a contemporary look. All of us need to periodically update our hairstyle, clothing, and accessories. Styles change. Appearance matters. If your look is outdated, people can't help wondering if your knowledge and skills are outdated too.

Work at getting and staying fit. This will boost your confidence, make you look and feel better, and improve your brainpower and stamina. Many fitness clubs and programs cater to those over age 55.

Stay actively engaged in learning. Some people become intimidated by new ways of doing things as they get older. But it's the best way to stay engaged in life. Learning keeps you young, makes you feel alive, and keeps you current with knowledge, information, and skills. There is even evidence that we lose less brain cells due to aging if we stay actively engaged in learning new things. It's never too late to go back to school for a higher degree or even just to take some courses. Remember, education is a gift you give yourself.

Stay upbeat, friendly, and easy-going. Maintain a sense of fun and colleagueship in your workplace. Don't keep to yourself or only associate with those in your own age bracket. Express interest in or learn something about popular culture (movies, musicians, fashion, trends) from your kids, grandkids, or coworkers.

Consider alternate work settings. There are many work settings and opportunities that offer less physically demanding work and a more regular schedule if that is what you are looking for. Consider the outpatient setting and community health, such as school nursing, public health, clinics, blood banks, adult day care, etc. There are also many nontraditional opportunities with insurance companies, private review companies, government and public agencies, and traditional healthcare facilities in specialties such as case management, telephone advice line, disease management, patient advocate, etc.

There are also some low-key positions for nurses to work in assisted living and rehabilitation facilities where you only give out medication to ambulatory or semiambulatory patients and do not need to provide any physical care or do any lifting.

Retiring

Retirement is a big life change. Even though some people look forward to this time of "leisure" in their lives, they often don't know what to do with themselves once they get there. Others initially enjoy traveling, spending time with family and friends, and engaging in leisure pursuits. But after a while, they long to be doing something more meaningful and constructive with their time. Some also want to continue to contribute to their community in some way. No one retires to a rocking chair on the porch anymore!

For nurses who do wish to retire — whether on a temporary, permanent or part-time (semiretirement) basis, there are several things you can do to stay connected to your profession. After all, nursing is not something you just turn off when you are no longer working. Many nurses experience a sense of loss or sadness when they retire and feel disconnected. But you don't have to keep working to stay connected to nursing or to contribute to your community.

It's important to stay mentally and physically active and engaged during retirement. It's fine to spend time with your grandkids, but you have to maintain your own interests, activities, leisure pursuits, and life. Here are some strategies to make the most of your retirement.

Stay connected through nursing professional associations. Even if you never belonged to anything before, join now. Consider joining your state nurses association and/or a specialty association that you can relate to. Most associations have reduced dues for retired members. Some even have "retired nurse" coalitions. If yours doesn't, start one. This is a great way to stay connected and informed, maintain a sense of colleagueship, and get involved in projects when and if you feel like it.

Consider part-time work. If you want to keep working, even occasionally, contact your city and county board of health and make yourself available (on a paid or volunteer basis) to give flu shots and vaccinations or work at health fairs and public screening clinics. Contact your local board of education to do substitute school nursing or to accompany frail children to school in districts that offer this service. You'll find education, counseling, and other client service positions available through social service agencies such as the American Red Cross, American Heart Association, Planned Parenthood, etc. You can also sign on with a nursing agency to be available on an occasional basis for many of the above things. This way you can stay loose with your commitments and work when and if you want to.

Consider volunteering. If you aren't necessarily interested in drawing a salary, consider volunteering in a healthcare setting. Many of the above settings offer volunteer opportunities. Also, schools and residences for the developmentally disabled look for "surrogate" or "foster" grandparents to come in and spend time with the kids. There are opportunities everywhere.

Enjoy! Whether you continue to work part-time, volunteer, or neither, this is the perfect time in your life to engage in artistic activities, develop a new hobby, or further your education. Some people work to fill a void in their life because that's all they've ever known. Yet there are so many other things to learn — about yourself and the world around you. Grandma Moses didn't start painting until she was in her 70s!

Special Situations

Returning to the Workforce

If you've been away from the nursing workforce for some years for whatever reason, there are a number of things that you can and should do to facilitate a smooth transition back. It can be unnerving to return to work. Most people feel unsure of themselves, lack confidence, and wonder if anyone will hire them. It is common to be uncertain about how to get started or where to look to get reconnected to their profession and to get up to date on trends, skills, and information. Here are steps to facilitate the process and build confidence.

1. Join and get active in your state nurses association. If you've been out of the workforce, this is a great way to get reconnected to your profession — even if you've never belonged before. It's also a great way to get current on what's happening in your profession.

2. Start volunteering. Since jumping right into a paid nursing position can be a bit unnerving, in addition to taking some time to find the right position, volunteering is a great way to ease your way back in. Volunteering will help you to build confidence, make valuable connections, hone old skills, and learn new ones. It will also give you recent relevant experience to put on your résumé and discuss in an interview. Besides all that, volunteering often leads to paid employment. So look for volunteer opportunities in settings where you'd ideally like to work or in a setting that feels comfortable. Consider any healthcare facility, social service agency, clinic, public health agency, or organization, etc.

3. Get out to career fairs and facility open houses. These events, advertised in local newspapers and nursing publications and websites, are great venues to "test the waters" and to see what is available. Attending these events is also a perfect way to brush up on your self-marketing and networking skills, which get rusty with disuse.

Returning to Bedside Nursing

If you are an experienced nurse who wishes to return to direct patient care in an acute (hospital), subacute, or long-term care setting after an extended absence (more than a few years), then a refresher course is probably in order. An "absence" here could mean that you've been out of the workforce or that you've worked in a different type of specialty, one where you did not deliver traditional hands-on care, such as case management, administration, and education, etc.

Since every employer is different, before enrolling in any courses, make some preliminary phone calls to the nurse recruiter in area healthcare facilities. Find out if you are eligible for hire at this point, or if you would need to take a refresher course. Inquire as to whether each facility has a reentry program for experienced nurses returning to the bedside.

If you do wish to, or need to, take a refresher course, look for one that offers a comprehensive mix of classroom and clinical time, complete with preceptor. Refresher courses are offered by healthcare facilities, educational institutions, and private companies. They run anywhere from three to six months in length and generally cost $1,000 and up. Contact your state nurses association, state board of nursing, and state hospital association to locate courses in your area. You can also do an Internet search for, "RN (or LPN) refresher courses in [your state]."

If you are returning to the workforce but do not wish to return to bedside nursing, you likely will not need to take a refresher course unless you wish to, or if it is required by your state board of nursing to reactivate your license.

Nurses with Disabilities

Whether you come into nursing with a disability or develop one along the way, you have plenty of options. As I've said repeatedly, there is something for everyone in this profession. Depending on your needs, interests, and experiences, there are opportunities to work from home, in office settings, in latex-free environments, and in inpatient care settings that are less physically demanding than many traditional hospital positions. There are also adaptive devices available for those with hearing, visual, and other needs. There is no obstacle that can't be overcome with persistence and determination.

Although the Americans with Disabilities Act prohibits a prospective employer from discriminating against someone because of a disability, it doesn't prevent someone from not hiring you without revealing his or her reasons. So you may need to be creative, flexible, and persistent with your approach to job finding.

. . . .

Many nurses have unique challenges to overcome.

. . . .

You are not obligated to mention any medical condition or disability on an interview unless you need special accommodation. However, if your disability is obvious, i.e., you walk with a cane, use a wheelchair, wear dark glasses, have a tremor, etc., you might consider saying something in passing to alleviate any concerns the employer might have about liability issues or your ability to do a job. For example, if you walk with a cane, you might nonchalantly say during the interview, "By the way, although I do use a cane to walk, I have no limitations on how long I can be on my feet — just in case you were wondering." Say this with a smile on your face to reassure the employer.

When networking and going on job interviews, focus on your experience, credentials, and skill set. Downplay any limitations or disabilities. Of course, if you will need special accommodation on the job, you will need to mention that at some point, but don't bring it up in the beginning. Give any prospective employer an opportunity to get to know you and to be "sold" on you and your background. Remember that when all is said and done, employers look for someone with a positive, upbeat, can-do personality. So "Wow" them with your charm, your excellent communication skills, and your enthusiasm and professionalism.

Overcoming a Difficult Past

Many nurses have unique challenges to overcome from their past such as substance abuse, serious illness, or departure from a previous job under less than ideal circumstances. Although challenging, you can work through any of these situations with a little patience, persistence, and determination. Here are some tips to help you get your career back on track.

Work on getting positive and motivated: A problematic past is likely to make you feel insecure, scared, nervous, and possibly even depressed. This can show through in your facial expressions, body language, and demeanor. I've seen it many times: someone who doesn't smile, makes limited eye contact, appears on the verge of tears, and looks generally scared and nervous. Any probing question about work history sends you into a panic.

While it is understandable that you will be uneasy and uncertain while job hunting and interviewing in this situation, it is important that you focus on your good experience, credentials, and education. Focus on your great skills and abilities and the contributions you can make. Listen to or read motivational material. Sometimes we have to hear these things from other people. Review the section on challenges to moving forward in Chapter 3 and utilize the recommendations there.

Be ready for tough questions: It is inevitable that a prospective employer will ask about your work history, especially if there are gaps or if your employment history is erratic. Be prepared with answers to questions you will likely be asked. In Chapter 7, I discussed how to address interview questions related to why you left your last job when there was a problem. In Chapter 8, I discussed how to address related issues on your résumé and cover letter.

Start out volunteering: When you have a problematic background, volunteering is an excellent way to ease your way back into the job market. It will give your day or week purpose and structure so that you don't dwell on your troubles. Too much time on your hands can play havoc with your psyche and lead to more depression and self-doubt. I discussed the benefits of volunteering earlier in this chapter in the section on returning to the workforce.

Do more networking: As already mentioned, networking is a great way to find a job, especially when you have obstacles to overcome. That means that you need to get yourself out amongst "the living." Get yourself a business suit or great business outfit and start attending career fairs, conventions, and association meetings. Let colleagues and friends know that you are looking for work and ask for help. It is always easier to get a job when you have someone make a recommendation, referral, or introduction for you.

Seek job assistance: Most state nurses associations have Peer Assistance programs for nurses in recovery from substance abuse. Contact your SNAs whether you are a member or not. Contact local community colleges about career counseling and seek the services of a career coach, preferably one who is a nurse. Don't try to go it alone. Utilize every resource that is available to you.

Give yourself a competitive edge: Join and get active in some professional associations. This shows you are an involved and informed member of your profession. Besides, this is one of the best ways to stay current with knowledge and trends. Enroll in some college courses and utilize online and live continuing education courses.

Additional Questions

Q: *What do I do if I get laid off from my job?*

A: Getting laid-off can be devastating. But it can also be the universe's way of telling you it's time to move on. Grieve your loss and take time to destress and unwind before launching a full-scale job search. A forced lapse in work is the perfect time to recharge your batteries and regroup before moving forward.

Develop a budget and see how long you can manage by living on your savings. Think of ways you can cut back on your expenditures if necessary. You'd be amazed at how little you can live on when necessary. Consider doing temp or agency work while you look for more permanent employment.

It is not wise to let your healthcare insurance coverage lapse, especially if you or a covered family member has a preexisting condition. If your employer provided you with healthcare benefits, you, and your covered dependents may be eligible under the Consolidated Omnibus Budget Reconciliation Act (COBRA) for temporary continuation of healthcare coverage at group rates. Under COBRA, you are responsible for paying the entire cost of the premium. Your employer should be able to provide you with more information about the rules and regulations that govern COBRA, or you can contact the U.S. Department of Labor at (866) 444-3272.

You may even be eligible for unemployment insurance, depending on the circumstances of your separation. Don't be ashamed or embarrassed to utilize any benefits you have coming to you.

Immediately activate your network of friends, associates, and colleagues. Get on the phone and out to networking events and let everyone know you're in the job market. Be sure to save your receipts, too, since your job hunting expenses may be tax deductible in this situation.

Q: *I was fired from my job but believe the firing was unjust. What recourse do I have?*

A: If you believe you were treated unfairly on a job and wrongly terminated, you have several courses of action that may be appropriate. Check your employer's policy on filing grievances. Take that tack if appropriate.

You can also check with your state department of labor (www.dol.gov). Representatives are available to offer advice and information on work-related issues.

Consider consulting a nurse attorney or any qualified attorney who specializes in employment law. You can find a nurse attorney through The American Association of Nurse Attorneys (www.taana.org) or from a referral through your state nurses association. (Go to www.nursingworld.org and click on "Constituent Member Associations.")

Q: *I've considered working for myself either as an entrepreneur, consultant, or independent contractor. How do I get started?*

A: There are many great opportunities for self-employment for nurses, and we make great business owners. Start by attending a related seminar and/or by taking business courses through a local community college. You'll also find some great books in the public library about business ownership, consulting, and related topics. For additional information and support, contact the U.S. Small Business Administration (www.sba.gov) and the National Nurses in Business Association (www.nnba.net).

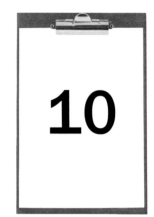

The Finishing Touches

Stop for a moment and reflect on where you are in your career and think about what you'd like to accomplish in the future. Perhaps you've been contemplating going back to school, getting certified in your specialty, or running for office in your professional association. You may even be thinking about doing more writing or speaking or transitioning into a management position. Thoughts, ideas, and dreams are great, but they don't create action — and action is what gets things done. There's no better way to create positive action in your life than setting goals.

Goals are your life's game plan. They state how you'll live, where you'll go, and how you will get there. They give you a purpose to work toward. They must be specific, exact things you want to accomplish. Everyone needs to have long- and short-term goals. A long-term goal is something you want to accomplish in the next five years; a short-term goal is something you want to accomplish in the next year or less. For example, your long-term goal is to graduate from college. The short-term goals are to research the schools offering the degree you want and to submit an application to the college of your choice.

Goals must be written down or they become day dreams. You need to look at them often. A goal must be specific, challenging, objective, measurable, and have a timeframe.

Here are some long- and short-term goals:

- Get an article published in a nursing journal within the next year
- Submit a proposal to speak at a nursing conference in the next six months
- Obtain clinical certification within the next three years
- Become a part-time CPR instructor in one year

Write down your goals perhaps on 3 X 5 index cards, each with an accompanying target date. Keep them where you will look at them often. This will keep you focused and on track. Research has shown that if you don't write down your goals, you're much less likely to act on them and more inclined to forget them. It serves as a visible reminder to get moving. When you reach a goal, cross it off, and set a new one. Stretch yourself; have purpose. That's what keeps life interesting.

To start you off, here are seven items for your 3 X 5 cards:

Learn High-Tech Etiquette

Since the mid-1990s, communicating has become both easier and more complicated. Today we can reach almost anyone at any time. We have become "communication junkies," addicted to our e-mail or cell phones. Many of us suffer withdrawal when we're away from them even for a short time. Stories of cell phone abuse are abundant, and e-mailing has generated new means of expression with emoticons and such. The rules, written and unwritten, for effective appropriate communication, have been evolving.

Voice Mail

Be prepared to speak to an answering machine or voice mail system. Know what you want to say so your message will be brief and concise. Don't ramble or speak rapidly. Enunciate clearly, giving your full name and phone number, including area code even if the other person already has it. This saves that person the time of looking it up when returning your call. Repeat your phone number a second time so the person doesn't have to keep replaying your message to get the number. It's also a good idea to mention when it would be a good time to reach you to minimize telephone tag.

When you are returning a stranger's call, jog the other person's memory by stating what their phone call was about (if you know). That person may have called a number of other people and might not immediately remember why they called you. For example, you might say, "This is Jordan Sparks returning your phone call. You left me a message inquiring about guidelines for continuing education credits."

Cell Phones

Cell phone usage spread faster than the flu. And while they are credited with saving many lives, they have also been blamed for car accidents, disrupted concerts, meetings, and meals. Of course the cell phone itself isn't the problem: It's the people who use them in inappropriate ways and places.

Here are some simple common sense rules to follow:

- You don't need to speak louder than normal on a cell phone; very few people are interested in your personal business.
- When using your cell phone in public places, avoid close proximity to other people whenever possible.
- Turn off your phone or set it to vibrate while in restaurants, libraries, during seminars/classes, performances, and places of worship.
- Never take calls during an interview (yes, this happens!), performance appraisal, or a negotiation. Unless you're expecting the birth of a child or are a high-ranking government official, things can wait until you pick up your voice mail messages. Set limits.

E-mail

Because it's fast and inexpensive, e-mail has become the primary means of communication for many people. Yet it is not appropriate in all circumstances and does not replace many traditional forms of communication. For example, an interview thank-you note, as mentioned in Chapter 8, should still be sent via the U.S. Postal Service snail mail in most cases. You should never resign from a job, discuss a sensitive subject, or respond in an angry way through e-mail. And since you don't have the benefit of nonverbal communication cues when using e-mail, choose your words carefully before hitting the send button.

As a reminder, here are some e-mail basics:

- **Be formal.** Write a work-related e-mail as if you were writing a letter or memo. Use proper grammar, punctuation, spelling, and salutations. Proofread the note before sending and don't rely exclusively on spell-check.
- **Include the sender's message.** With all the e-mail correspondence sent today, it's impossible to recall what you said to whom. So make sure you include the sender's message when you reply to an e-mail. I've received e-mail responses that said, "Yes. That's great." I had no idea what the person was responding to, so I had to go into my "sent" file and search for my last e-mail to them, if I even saved it. It's time-consuming and annoying.
- **Consider skipping attachments.** Because of all the computer viruses circulating today, don't send an attachment unless it's something impor-

tant and to someone whom you've told to expect it. Otherwise, you run the risk of having your message deleted without being read. And larger attachments run the risk of not going through at all.

- **Use a clear subject line.** Giving receivers an idea about the content of your e-mail ensures that they'll know if they need to read your e-mail immediately. Avoid generic subject phrases like, "Hi." If the subject changes after several messages, change the subject line, too.

Faxes

Use a cover sheet that clearly indicates who the fax is to and from and how many pages you are sending. If some pages do not get properly transmitted, the receiver might not realize they are missing anything if they don't know how many pages you intended to send. Don't send lengthy documents (more than 5 pages) via fax unless you've been asked to do so. Anything more than that ties up the receiver's fax machine, has a tendency to jam at one end or the other, and uses up a lot of paper on the receiving end. If you have a multipage document to send, consider mailing it via the U.S. Postal Service.

Technology can be a great tool when used appropriately. However, you'll lose credibility and miss out on many opportunities when it becomes obvious that you haven't learned the rules. Boost your image, your workplace savvy, and your effectiveness by learning and using communication technology in a considerate and responsible way.

Have Business Cards Made

Every nurse needs to have a business card. Why? Because this is how professional people network and exchange contact information. Many nurses are under the mistaken impression that "business cards" are only for those who own a business. On the contrary, they are simply "calling cards" used for professional networking. Today, anyone who's anybody has a business card, and every nurse is definitely somebody. Business cards are a professional way of introducing yourself. They create the opportunity to stay in touch with people. People exchange business cards with one another in both social and workplace situations. Besides, having a business card makes you feel important.

If you already have a card from your place of employment, that's fine. However, you may want to have your own cards made with personal contact information on them. This way, people can get in touch with you outside of work and can still reach you if you ever leave your current job. Many of us change jobs more often than we move our place of residence. Of course, you can always write your personal information on the back of your work-related card so that people feel like they're getting special access to you.

If you don't have work-related cards, ask your supervisor if you can get them. Explain they are part of your professional image when you are representing your employer, and that you need them for professional networking both in and outside of your place of employment. Be prepared to sell the idea. It's worth a try. In fact, many nurses who have work-related business cards hand them out to patients and their families in certain circumstances. You have to decide if that's appropriate for you.

In any event, you can have your own cards made easily and inexpensively at any local print shop. And while it is possible to print business cards on your personal computer, it's not recommended because the card stock is flimsy, and the design, layout, and print will not have a truly professional look to it. Your business card makes a statement about you and is part of your professional image. It's a self-marketing tool. Your business card should not appear cheap or homemade. It should convey style and professionalism.

Start with a white card with black lettering for maximum impact. For a professional look, avoid graphics such as flowers, etc. Be sure the type size and font style is easily readable. Ask the printer for recommendations and examples.

Frequently Asked Questions

Q: *What information should be on my personal business card?*

A: Start with your name followed by professional credentials. Include your address, phone number, fax number, and e-mail address (see example). Remember, you won't be giving cards that list your personal information to patients. You'll be using them for professional networking.

Phone: 555-222-4545

Janet Fredericks, RN, MS

22 Elm Street   janet@net.net
Essex, NJ 09988   Fax: 555-222-4444

Q: *How should I list my initials after my name on my business card?*

A: This is an age-old question. While some people list their nursing credentials first and their degrees second, either way is correct. Those in academic circles prefer the college degree first and the nursing credential second. After that, list your certifications and special affiliations. Here are some examples:

Karen Collins, RN, PhD, FAAN
Karen Collins, PhD, RN, FAAN

Robert Allen, RN, MS, CNOR
Katherine Caldwell, BSN, RN

Q: *Should I list my ADN? If I get an MSN, should I drop the BSN?*

A: If you have multiple degrees in varying majors, it is most practical to simply list the highest degree earned. If you have both an MBA and an MSN for example, you might simply use the MSN or list both depending on the environment you work in. Don't get carried away with initials. This is just a calling card, not a bio sketch.

Q: *Should I list things like, "CPR certified" or some sort of title or specialty under my name?*

A: It is not necessary or advisable to list credentials like BLS (Basic Life Support) or ACLS (Advanced Cardiac Life Support) on your business card. It is also not necessary to list something like, "Psychiatric nurse," or, "Oncology nurse," under your name, unless you are promoting a consulting practice in that specialty.

Q: *Who needs business cards?*

A: Every nurse and student nurse needs a card whether actively working, retired, between jobs, a full-time student, currently out of the workforce for any reason, etc. No one is exempt.

Q: *How and when would I use a business card?*

A: Once you have business cards, you'll be amazed at all the practical uses and opportunities that exist to exchange contact information. Here are just a few examples:

- Enclose your card when mailing a gift, photo, article, or résumé to someone.

- Exchange cards with colleagues you meet at association meetings, seminars, or conventions so you can stay in touch with them for support and information sharing.

- Present your card when meeting a key media person, author, or industry leader and offer yourself as a resource for future programs/articles.

- Offer your card to someone from a company you always wanted to work for. Ask them to keep you in mind if anything comes up.

- Enclose your card when sending a card or handwritten note to someone so the person can get in touch with you if he or she wishes.

- Give your card to those you mentor or precept. This way they'll be able to get in touch with you when they need to.

- Provide your card to someone who offers to send you some information.

Use Them!

Once you have business cards made, carry them with you wherever you go. Don't leave them in your office, in your car, at home, or in your hotel room when at a conference. I always have a few business cards with me no matter where I go — and that includes the beach, on vacation, to the beauty parlor, and to social events. You never know whom you'll meet where, and you always want to be prepared.

To add an extra element of style, get a business card holder to carry in your pocket or purse. This is a small pouch or hinged box. Not only does it make a great presentation, but it keeps your cards from getting dog-eared and dirty. Your card is part of your professional image so keep them clean and up to date. If information changes, get new cards made. Don't cross out the old information and pen in the new info. That's tacky and unprofessional.

Be sure your cards are readily accessible so you don't have to start digging in your purse or wallet to find one. If you're attending a networking event, put a handful of cards in your pocket or other easily accessible place so you can retrieve one with ease. Some people keep their own cards in one pocket, and those they collect from others in another.

Q: *Is there a proper way to present my card or ask people for theirs?*

A: Yes! Distribute your cards with discretion. Don't hand them out as if you were dealing out a poker hand. And don't thrust it into someone's hand when you first meet him. Rather, it is appropriate to engage in some conversation with someone before offering your card. Then say something like, "May I give you my card?" or, "I'd like to give you my card." You can add, "Please feel free to call on me if I can help you in any way." Or, "Keep me in your Rolodex and use me as a resource," or, "Perhaps we can talk further after today and share some information." When presenting your card, hand it print side up and facing the receiver so they can read it without turning it.

If someone asks you for your card, and you don't have one with you, don't ever say, "I don't have a card; but if you give me one of yours, I'll write my name and number on the back." Some people find that tacky and offensive. Just because you don't have a card doesn't give you the right to use theirs as scrap paper. Rather, write your name and contact information on a piece of paper or offer to send your card to them when you get home. Of course the exception would be if someone offers you his or her own business card for that express purpose. A better solution is to never be caught without your cards.

When requesting someone else's card, say something like, "May I have your business card?" or, "Do you have a business card?" When accepting someone else's business card, it is polite to look it over for a moment and comment on it. Make note of their name, title, and organization if applicable. You might say, "I see you're located in New York City. Have you been there long?" If it is a workplace card, you might say their title out loud and comment, "What exactly does a Director of Patient Care Services do?" You can also say something like, "May I call on you in the future if I have further questions?"

Once you have your business cards, you're ready to move forward.

Firm Up Your Handshaking Technique

If you want to be taken seriously as a nurse, you need to start shaking hands. Handshaking is an important social custom in the western world. Extending your hand to someone is a sign of respect. Proper handshaking will enhance your credibility and put you, along with the entire profession, on a more equal footing with other professions in healthcare and society in general.

The handshake is an important part of a first impression. In many situations, people will evaluate you based on whether or not you shake hands and the quality of your handshake. A limp handshake may give the impression that you are an insecure or insincere person, while a firm handshake conveys character and authority. I've already mentioned how important the handshake is on a job interview and in networking situations, but there are many other occasions when a handshake should be used as well.

It is particularly important for nurses to shake hands with their patients and patients' families when appropriate. Obviously it would not be appropriate in emergency situations but can be used in many healthcare settings and situations. As caregivers, nurses have license to have physical contact with others that goes beyond what is usually socially acceptable. Therefore, initially shaking hands with a patient during an introduction is a respectful way of starting the care giving relationship. It is also a good chance for the patient and nurse to start creating a bond of trust. Likewise, a nurse should shake hands with family members, physicians, and other healthcare professionals as well as colleagues that you do not see on a regular basis, such as those you see at meetings and conventions.

How to Shake Hands

There are many wrong ways to shake hands but only one right way. Approach the person with whom you wish to shake hands. Maintain eye contact with the other person and, when you're about three feet away, fully extend your right hand with your thumb pointing up. Engage the other person's hand, making palm to palm contact, locking thumb webs. Your fingers should wrap around the other person's hand in a firm grip (don't crush the other person's metacarpals). Then use one or two downward pumps and release the grip, all while maintaining eye contact.

Be sure to smile while you're at it, conveying confidence, warmth, and sincerity. It's a three pronged approach: a full firm handshake, eye contact, and a smile. A handshake without eye contact is not considered credible. You will encounter some less than desirable handshakes such as the "dead fish" or "fingertips only." Remain steady with your own firm handshake. You cannot control the other person's handshake; you can only control your own.

If someone is standing and offers to shake your hand, you should stand to shake theirs, whether you are a man or a woman. This promotes a sense of equality in some cases and respect between the parties. Although a handshake would not "equalize" the relationship between an older person and a younger person or a senior person and a junior person in a corporation, it can make a statement that both parties are important in their unique roles. This could be the case with nurses shaking hands with physicians and other healthcare professionals, for example.

What Not to Do

Just as there is an appropriate way to shake hands, there are some things to avoid:

- Avoid a two-handed shake in which people use their second hand to cover the clasped hands or to enclose the other person's one hand in their two hands. Although often done as a friendly gesture, people can misconstrue this handshake technique as motherly, controlling, or too intimate.

There is a natural and legitimate concern amongst nurses about the transmission of germs by hand to hand contact. However, the opportunity to connect with another person through a respectful form of touching outweighs the potential drawbacks. And good hygiene, including frequent hand washing and the regular use of waterless sanitizer, will minimize any infection control issues.

- Do not put your free hand on the other person's shoulder or grip his or her forearm while shaking hands. By so doing, you step beyond what is socially acceptable and invade his or her personal space.

- Pause for a moment before pulling your hand out of the shake. Try to be the last person to release the grip. It may seem awkward at first, but you'll get a feel for it with some experience.

- If you pour cologne or perfume into your hands to pat on your face or pulse points, be sure to wash your hands well afterwards. You don't want everyone you shake hands with to smell you on their hands for the rest of the day.

When to Shake Hands

Now that you know the proper way to shake hands, when is it appropriate to shake? A handshake should always be used —

- Upon meeting someone for the first time

- To greet someone you don't see on a regular basis

- At the start and end of an interview, even if you know the person well

- When parting company with those you just met and/or don't see often

- After a meeting or conversation to show agreement or solidarity

- Whenever someone offers his or her hand to you

- When you're welcoming people into your home, your office, or a meeting

Troubleshooting

Even with the best of intentions, there are often obstacles and stumbling blocks to something as seemingly simple as a handshake. They might include —

- **Being unable to shake hands.** If, for example, you've had recent hand surgery or have severe arthritis, you might politely say something like, "Forgive me for not shaking your hand, but I recently had hand surgery."

• •

I like to shake hands with members of my audience when I am giving a presentation — either before or after the event. It's a good way to introduce yourself, make attendees feel special, and to make a more personal connection with audience members.

• •

• **Having cold hands or sweaty palms.** Shake anyway. The receiver is probably much less aware of the state of your hand than you are. Don't apologize for your cold or sweaty hands and draw attention to them. Of course, if you know beforehand that you will be greeting someone and shaking hands, you can prepare. If your hands are cold, rub them together when no one is looking. If you have sweaty palms, keep a handkerchief in your pocket and use it discreetly, if possible, just before shaking to dry off your hand. If that's not feasible, shake hands anyway. The act of shaking hands is more important than the fact that your hand is sweaty or cold. If you refuse to shake, people may assume that you are unfriendly or do not respect them. Refusing to shake someone's extended hand is insulting unless you offer an acceptable reason, such as religious proscription or physical limitation.

• •

People with Disabilities

Just because someone has a disability, it doesn't mean you should bypass the traditional handshake. This convention is important with people who are disabled and who are often marginalized or treated differently. As nurses, we have a responsibility to be role models for greetings and behaviors that are respectful and appropriate for all people, especially those with a physical or mental disability.

If someone is visually impaired, you might ask, "May I shake your hand?" and then bring your hand to meet his or hers. If someone has a missing or nonfunctioning right hand or limb, offer your left hand to shake. Likewise, if someone offers the left hand first for whatever reason, meet it with your left. If someone has limited use of both limbs, extend your right hand anyway close to his or her right hand. People with a limitation will usually make an effort to meet your hand in some capacity. If shaking isn't possible, a nod of the head or a light touch on the hand is appropriate to acknowledge the person.

• •

Cultural Differences

Cultural differences exist where handshaking and eye contact are concerned, and it is important for nurses to be aware of some of the differences. While it is common for those from Europe and Australia to shake hands and make direct eye contact, it is much less common in those from Asian countries where less eye contact and a more delicate handshake might be the preferred norm. This does not mean that you must adapt your handshake depending on someone's country of origin. It simply means that you should be aware that differences exist so that you do not misinterpret someone else's habits or behaviors.

Also some men of orthodox Jewish faith and Muslim faith are not permitted to have physical contact with a woman other than a close family member. So how do you know who to extend your hand to and who not to? In some cases, you can identify a man of orthodox Jewish faith by his distinctive dress. With that exception, it is better to extend your hand in most situations as a gesture of good will. If the other person cannot shake hands for religious reasons, they will usually graciously state, "My culture does not permit me to shake hands," or something similar. In that case you would simply drop your hand back to your side and nod a greeting. There is no reason for embarrassment or feelings of being slighted.

- **Getting brushed off.** If you extend your hand to someone to shake, and he or she does not respond, simply drop your hand to your side and carry on. Who knows what his or her motivation is. Just don't take it personally.

- **Having your hands full (literally).** If you're holding something in your right hand when someone approaches you to shake hands, put whatever it is down or shift it to your left hand. At networking and social events, carry a drink in your left hand so you are prepared to shake hands. You can also extend your left hand, if necessary, in a pinch.

Proper handshaking conveys confidence, trust, and openness. If you already have a good, firm handshake and use it regularly, you're ahead of the game. If not, start practicing to perfect your grip and begin using your newly acquired skill.

Brush Up on Your Conversational Skills

"Don't talk to strangers," is the warning we grew up with. So it's natural to feel uncomfortable striking up a conversation with people you don't know. Most of us are reluctant to walk up to strangers and introduce ourselves. But if you work to overcome this, you will have the social advantage. Here are some strategies that work.

If you find yourself at an event with no one to talk to, look for someone who also appears to be alone rather than trying to break into a group discussion. If you use your observational skills, you'll get a sense of who is open to talking versus those who seem to want to be alone. If you approach someone who won't make eye contact or smile and who seems distracted or disinterested, just move on. You might also approach the food table, if there is one, and say to someone there, "This looks good. Do they always put out this kind of spread?"

Be observant and find something to compliment like a piece of jewelry, a tie, or article of clothing. Most of us appreciate a sincere compliment, and often there's a story associated with the item like a great vacation or holiday. Now you've started a light conversation.

I've had interesting conversation with people I've encountered on airplanes and in the beauty parlor by commenting on a book they were reading or carrying. You might say, "I noticed you are reading Toni Morrison's latest book, and I was thinking of buying it. Are you enjoying it?" There are opportunities to network virtually everywhere.

If you're attending a seminar or workshop, you might ask fellow attendees on a break, "How do you like the program so far?" or, "Where did you travel from today?" These are easily answered icebreakers that invite further conversation. They open the door for you to introduce yourself and extend your hand for a handshake. Many people will welcome your initiative with a sigh of relief for getting the ball rolling. Warming up with an icebreaker or two makes self-introduction much less intimidating.

How do you keep the ball rolling once you get it going? It's always a good idea to stay focused on the other person by showing interest in them and what they do. It's said that everyone's favorite subject to talk about is him- or herself. Ask a few simple "yes" or "no" or open ended questions such as, "Are you a member of this association? For how long? What do like about it?" Be sure to offer like information about yourself, too, without monopolizing the conversation. Networking is a reciprocal give and take relationship. It's only through self-disclosure that you'll reap the maximum benefit.

• •

If you're feeling out of the loop and not up on what's happening in the world, read a weekly news magazine before going out. These publications usually provide a good overview of world events; domestic news; pop culture; and the latest book, movie, and music releases.

• •

Avoid the "hot" topics like politics, religion, and anything you're passionate about where you can't tolerate another opinion. Safe topics of conversation are the weather, certain current events, sports and entertainment, and industry issues. If you're sitting at a table with others, you might say, "Did anyone see the news story about (fill in the blank)?" or, "Has anyone seen the movie (fill in the blank)?" Choose a topic in which you're interested or have some expertise. With some practice, you will overcome your shyness and fear of talking to people.

Finding a Mentor

There is an abundance of material on how to be a good mentor but very little is written on how to find one. How can you find the right person to advise, guide, and coach you? And how do you approach that person once you do find them? Consider these points.

Getting Started

Think about what you want to accomplish before contacting a potential mentor. Are you looking to advance in your current place of employment, succeed in a new job, or do you simply want to be better in your chosen specialty? A mentor can be helpful in a variety of situations and in various phases of your career. However, experienced nurses who want to make the move to the next level or make a change within their career often benefit most from being mentored.

What to Look For

When considering a potential mentor, look for someone who you admire and respect. It is also important to find someone who is experienced and successful in their profession or specialty, not to mention well connected. Likewise, it is advantageous to seek out someone who seems approachable and friendly and who is passionate and enthusiastic about their work; in other words, someone you would feel comfortable with.

Where to Look

Someone who is self-employed or who works for a different employer than you do is more likely to be your mentor. But don't overlook someone who works with you. Consider a current or former instructor or someone who holds a position you aspire to as a mentor, even if they are retired. Some professional associations have mentoring programs that match experienced colleagues with up and coming members.

How to Initiate the Relationship

Make a list of all the people you know who fit the preceding descriptions. Has any one of them shown an interest in you and your career? Has anyone been particularly helpful? Possibly you're surrounded by potential mentors, people giving you advice and guidance. You need to take the lead and see if any of them are willing to develop a more formal relationship.

In some cases, it's better to let the relationship develop naturally. Perhaps you've been getting occasional advice from a former supervisor or instructor. Maybe there is someone who you simply know or admire. Contact that person and let them know how much you respect them and value their opinion and that you aspire to be more like them. Ask if you could meet with them for 20 to 30 minutes to learn more about them. You should then begin to develop a sense of the person's comfort and the potential for a more formal relationship with you.

You may need or want to approach someone who does not know you. In this case, you might initially send a letter of introduction expressing your interest in speaking with that person, noting that you will call them as follow-up. Express your interest in that person and your value of their experience. Once you have met and established a relationship, ask if he or she would be willing to mentor you to work toward achieving your career goals.

Keep in mind that some people simply do not have the time or energy to be a mentor, so don't take it personally if that is the response you get. Maintain a relationship with that person anyway and look for another prospective mentor.

How to Be a Good Protégé

All relationships are two-way; both parties must benefit. Your mentor will benefit from your feedback regarding his or her advice, both good and bad. Always keep your mentor posted on your progress. Support your mentor in several ways, such as nominating him or her for awards. Always be ready to show your appreciation by referring potential clients or by passing on information and resources that may be of interest to them, if appropriate.

Some Additional Things to Consider

Can your boss be your mentor? It's possible but not ideal. The need to discuss sometimes sensitive workplace issues and on the job politics and competition favors a mentor to whom you don't report. Also, you needn't be of the same gender or in the same specialty as your mentor.

All relationships change over time, so you are likely to have several mentors over the course of your career. Don't take the hard road and do things on your own. Most successful people were guided and supported by mentors. Seek these people out for success.

Put Yourself First

The critical flaw in caregiving is that care for the caregiver often has the lowest priority. Airline passengers are cautioned, in an emergency, that they should put their oxygen masks on first before helping others. That is because if they become incapacitated, then they are of no use to themselves or others. Nurses are professional caregivers. We can see firsthand the effects of having little time and energy for ourselves: Stress, illness, short tempers, loss of focus and perspective, poor judgment, and errors. When you are overtaxed, things start to go wrong. It's impossible to avoid stress, but you can fight its effects.

Find Respite in Your Day

The more extended your nonstop efforts become, the less effective you may be, and the more likely you may be to make mistakes. How many nurses regularly skip breaks and meals? It is imperative to pause for recovery and renewal, even if for a few minutes at a time. Shift your focus to other matters by stepping outside, sitting in a chapel or meditation room, or taking a few deep breaths in another quiet spot.

Rediscover Yourself

A frantic pace in everyday life can sweep away our sense of self. When I ask nurses what they enjoy doing, some cannot answer the question because it's been so long since they did anything for fun. They have become so unaccustomed to having free time with activities of their own.

Try journaling, creating self-portrait collages (cutting out words, images, and symbols from magazines that you identify with and pasting them on poster board), and listening to music from your youth can help you regain a sense of self. Spend time with a hobby, take up an artistic pursuit, commune with nature. Balance the demands of our profession by creating a full, satisfying life outside of work.

Get Physical

The Greek philosopher Aristotle described humans as psychosomatic, or mind/body entities. For either to function well, both mind and body need to be healthy; they are the two inseparable parts of the whole person. Exercise lowers stress, improves health, controls weight, elevates mood, and more. Nurses know this but ignore it too often. It is as if they think they're exempt from the advice they give their patients. And don't think being busy all day equates exercise; it doesn't by a long shot.

A daily walking routine is a good way to start, combining exercise with time to be alone with your thoughts. Some of us will find that a health club or fitness center suits us better. Exercise alone or get a workout buddy or two. You'll find yourselves sharing and venting as you walk, jog, or stretch together. Dancing, cycling, and swimming are great pursuits to invigorate the body, clear the mind, and work off the day's travails.

Use Relaxation Techniques

Think of yourself as a reservoir of mental and physical energy that needs to be refilled before running dry. Meditation, stretching, and deep breathing will refill the reservoir and rejuvenate the spirit. They can be done virtually anywhere. They are more widely practiced today, and loads of books and articles on all three topics have been written to guide you in proper techniques. Don't overlook the benefits of massage, Reiki, and acupressure. These are necessities, not luxuries, for easing tension and tight muscles, and for realigning physical and mental energy. Ask for gift certificates to salons and spas for birthdays and holidays. Don't wait; treat yourself now because relaxation is routine maintenance for the mind, body, and spirit.

Care for the caregiver is top priority to ensure you can take care of everyone else with the focus, stamina, and enthusiasm they deserve.

Create a Professional Image

Last but certainly not least is the subject of appearance and image. While we've already discussed the importance of appearance on a job interview, your appearance and overall image will be a major factor in your future success — or lack of it. Having a license, credentials, and experience are simply not enough to convey professionalism and character. You have to look the part of a professional nurse as well as be the part. You have to inspire confidence in others. Simply put, you have to develop a professional image to match the professional person you are.

Whether you work in a hospital, office, corporate setting, or in the field, your appearance matters. Your clothing, your grooming, and your accessories make a loud statement about who you are and what you stand for. And as a professional nurse, you represent your entire profession whenever you interact with others.

First impressions and overall image impact our professional and personal lives every day in every situation. Nonverbal communication accounts for more than half of the message you send out when interacting with people. Like it or not, people judge us based on our appearance just as we do with others.

Whether you wear scrubs, uniforms, business casual clothes, or business suits, you should always be conservatively and meticulously attired and groomed in workplace and professional settings. In the movie *Working Girl,* actor Melanie Griffith, while trying to rise above her dead-end job, realizes that she has to change her image if she wants to get ahead. She utters the line, "If you want to be taken seriously, you need serious hair." You also need "serious" clothes and "serious" accessories.

In summary, whether happy in your current position, unemployed, or looking to make a change, it is vital to always be moving forward in your career. To make positive changes and create momentum in your professional life, you don't have to take a big leap of faith or make radical changes. Rather, you can start making small changes today, putting one foot in front of the other, moving forward in a positive direction. Move forward in faith and enjoy the journey!

I want to hear from you after you've finished reading this book. Please write to me and let me know how you used the information and the strategies provided. Tell me about your career and about lessons you've learned, rewards, and challenges, etc. I look forward to hearing from you!

Donna Cardillo, RN, MA
PO Box 15
Sea Girt, NJ 08750
donna@dcardillo.com

Resources

Recommended Reading

Cardillo, D. *Your First Year as a Nurse — Making the Transition from Total Novice to Successful Professional.* New York, NY: Three Rivers Press; 2001.

Fuimano, J. *The Journey Called You: A Roadmap to Self-Discovery and Acceptance.* Blue Bell, PA: Nurturing Your Success; 2005.

Borgatti J. *Frazzled, Fried...Finished? A Guide to Help Nurses Find Balance.* Bangor, ME: Booklocker.com; 2004.

Miller T. *Building and Managing a Career in Nursing — Strategies for Advancing Your Career.* Indianapolis, IN: Sigma Theta Tau International, Center for Nursing; 2002.

Maheady DC. *Leave No Nurse Behind: Nurses Working with disAbilities.* Lincoln, NE: iUniverse, Inc; 2006.

Sullivan EJ. *Becoming Influential — A Guide for Nurses.* Upper Saddle River, NJ: Prentice Hall; 2003.

Pagana K. *The Nurses Etiquette Advantage — How Professional Etiquette Can Advance Your Nursing Career.* Indianaplis, IN: Sigma Theta Tau International, Center for Nursing; 2008.

Bolles R. *What Color is Your Parachute?* Berkeley, CA: Ten Speed Press; 2008.

Johnson S, Blanchard K. *Who Moved My Cheese? An Amazing Way to Deal With Change in Your Work and in Your Life.* New York, NY: G. P. Putnam's Sons; 1998.

Sher B. *Wishcraft — How to Get What You Really Want.* New York, NY: Ballantine; 2003.

Richardson C. *Take Time for Your Life.* New York, NY: Broadway; 1999.

DVDs/CDs

Career Alternatives for Nurses® home study program on DVD and CD, by Donna Cardillo, RN.

Index

About the Author

Donna Wilk Cardillo, RN, MA, is the country's foremost authority on career development for nurses. She travels the world helping nurses to be happy in their careers and to reach their full potential. She is fiercely passionate about nursing and about life in general.

Donna is known as Dear Donna at *Nursing Spectrum* and *NurseWeek* magazines, where she writes a monthly column and doles out daily online career advice on nurse.com. Donna is the former Healthcare Careers Expert at monster.com

Donna is also author of *Your First Year as a Nurse — Making the Transition from Total Novice to Successful Professional.* She is creator of the Career Alternatives for Nurses® seminar and home study program.

Donna has received numerous awards and recognitions, but she is most proud of being named a Diva in Nursing by the Institute for Nursing in New Jersey for outstanding achievements and excellence in practice.

Donna is a life-long New Jersey resident — an original "Jersey Girl." She lives "down the shore" in Sea Girt, NJ, with her husband Joe.